Dignity in Care for Older People

Dignity in Care for Older People

Edited by

Lennart Nordenfelt

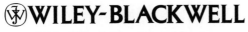

A John Wiley & Sons, Ltd., Publication

This edition first published 2009
© 2009 by Blackwell Publishing Ltd

Blackwell Publishing was acquired by John Wiley & Sons in February 2007. Blackwell's publishing programme has been merged with Wiley's global Scientific, Technical, and Medical business to form Wiley-Blackwell.

Registered office
John Wiley & Sons Ltd, The Atrium, Southern Gate, Chichester, West Sussex, PO19 8SQ, United Kingdom

Editorial offices
9600 Garsington Road, Oxford, OX4 2DQ, United Kingdom
2121 State Avenue, Ames, Iowa 50014-8300, USA

For details of our global editorial offices, for customer services and for information about how to apply for permission to reuse the copyright material in this book please see our website at www.wiley.com/wiley-blackwell.

Library of Congress Cataloging-in-Publication Data

Dignity in care for older people / edited by Lennart Nordenfelt.
    p. ; cm.
    Includes bibliographical references and index.
    ISBN 978-1-4051-8342-0 (pbk. : alk. paper)   1. Aged–Medical care.   2. Dignity.   3. Quality of life.   I. Nordenfelt, Lennart, 1945–
    [DNLM: 1. Geriatrics–ethics.   2. Health Services for the Aged–ethics.   3. Aged–psychology.
4. Personal Autonomy.   5. Quality of Life.   WT 21 D585 2009]

    RA564.8.D543 2009
    613'.0438–dc22

                                                                            2008053121

A catalogue record for this book is available from the British Library.

Set in 9.5 on 11.5 pt Palatino by SNP Best-set Typesetter Ltd., Hong Kong
Printed and bound in Malaysia by KHL Printing Co Sdn Bhd

1   2009

Contents

Contents

Contents

Preface

For several decades the concept of 'quality of life' has been well established in ethical debate about health care and the care of older people. There has been a growing concern among professionals involved in health care and the care of older people that the ultimate goal of care should not simply be to cure disease and forestall death. Instead, the general quality of life must be the main focus, whether the person concerned is ill or otherwise disabled. Quality of life is therefore often described as a significant separate goal both of ordinary medical care and of the care of older people. There has also been a concern that the care should be in accordance with certain basic ethical requirements. Thus the notions of autonomy and integrity have been highlighted. The autonomy and integrity of the patient or client, it has been claimed, must be respected in all instances.

The notion of dignity as a significant element in health-care discourse is more recent, but it has gradually acquired a more central place and is to be found in international conventions in the bioethical area, for instance the Council of Europe's *Bioethics Convention* (1997) and Unesco's *Universal Declaration on the Genome and Human Rights* (1997). In the latter document it is stated that 'research on the human genome ... should fully respect human dignity, freedom and human rights'. Dignity has also found a place in national legislation in the area of health care. An example is the most recent version of the Swedish Health and Medical Services Act (1997). In s. 2 of the Act it says: 'Care shall be given with respect for the equal value of all human beings and for the dignity of the individual.'

This book has as its main object of study the concept of dignity and its place in health and social care and especially the care of older people. The book has two concrete points of departure. These are two research projects, one supported by the European Commission, called Dignity and Older Europeans (DOE) (funded by the European Commission, DG Research, Directorate E: Biotechnology, Agriculture and Food, under FP5, Quality of Life Programme. Contract Number QLG6-CT-2001-00888) and one supported by the Swedish Vardal Foundation for Health Care Sciences and Allergy Research, called *Hemmet som den sista vårdplatsen* (literally, The Home as the Last Place of Care, called the Home project throughout this book). The focus in both these projects was on the situation and care of older people.

Before the two projects started, a number of theoretical studies with regard to the basic concepts of quality of life and dignity had been pursued. A subjective concept of quality of life, focusing on the notion of happiness, is briefly summarised in Chapter 1.

Preface

In the DOE project and in a few of the Home project studies, the four-notion dignity model (described in Chapter 2) served as a theoretical basis for individual and focus group interviews.

In the DOE project the focus groups had three target populations: older people themselves, professionals engaged in the care of older people, and young and middle-aged adults. All these interviews were collected and commented upon in summary reports issued by the DOE group. In the Home project the four-notion model functioned as a tool for the analysis of some of the empirical data from individual interviews.

All the authors of this book were connected either with the Home project or with the DOE project. We all hope that the material presented here may help in the education of health-care personnel, especially those involved in the care of older people.

Lennart Nordenfelt
Linköping, November 2008

Contributors

Jennifer Bullington is senior lecturer, Ersta Sköndal University College, Department of Health Care Sciences, Stockholm, Sweden. Her academic background is in philosophy and psychology and her clinical background is as a body-oriented psychotherapist. Her research is concerned mainly with phenomenology and psychosomatics. Some recent publications are: 'Body and self: a phenomenological study on the aging body and identity', *Medical Humanities* 32 (2006); M. Lundberg, J. Styf & J. Bullington, 'Experiences of moving with persistent pain – a qualitative study from a patient perspective', *Physiotherapy Theory and Practice* 23 (2007).

Michael Calnan is professor of medical sociology, University of Kent, Canterbury, UK. Calnan is a medical sociologist and has worked in health policy and health services research and training for over 20 years. His recent books include *Work Stress: The Making of a Modern Epidemic* (2002); and *Trust Matters in Health Care* (2008). His current research interests include diffusion and innovation in health care and technology, trust and health care, and dignity and the provision of health and social care for older people.

Ingrid Hellström has a background in gerontology nursing. She is senior lecturer and researcher at the Department of Palliative Care Research, Ersta Sköndal University College, Stockholm, Sweden. Her main research interest is older people with dementia and their spouses. Among her publications are: I. Hellström, M. Nolan & U. Lundh, 'Sustaining "couplehood". Spouses' strategies for living positively with dementia', *Dementia: The International Journal of Social Research and Practice* 6 (2007); and I. Hellström, M. Nolan, L. Nordenfelt & U. Lundh, 'Ethical and methodological issues in interviewing persons with dementia', *Nursing Ethics* 14 (2007).

Göran Lantz is consulting professor emeritus in health-care ethics, Uppsala University and Ersta Sköndal University College, Department of Health Care Sciences, Stockholm, Sweden. His research focus is in applied ethics, especially health-care ethics. Among his publications are: *Eigentumsrecht – ein Recht oder ein Unrecht?* [Property right – a right or a wrong?] Acta Universitatis Upsaliensis, Uppsala Studies in Social Ethics, 4 (1977), and *Vårdetik – berättelsen om Arthur* [Health-care ethics – the story of Arthur] (1992).

Lennart Nordenfelt is professor of philosophy of medicine and health care at Linköping University, Sweden. His main research interests lie within action theory, philosophy of medicine and health-care ethics. He has published works dealing with several basic medical concepts such as health, disability and health-care need. Among his publications are: *On the Nature of Health* (second, revised, edition 1995); and *Rationality and Compulsion* (2007).

Magnus Öhlander is associate professor in European Ethnology at Södertörn University College, Sweden. Among his research areas are geriatric care and health care in general, mainly with a focus on cultural aspects and ethnic relations. One of his publications is the article 'Problematic patienthood, "immigrants" in Swedish healthcare', *Ethnologia Scandinavica* 34 (2004). Recently he also published, together with O. Pripp, the book *Fallet Nogger Black: Antirasismens gränser* [The case of Nogger Black: the limits of anti-racism].

Win Tadd is senior research fellow, Department of Geriatric Medicine, Cardiff University, UK. Tadd's current research interests focus on the ethical aspects of ageing and care of older people, quality of care, long-term care and dignity and the provision of health and social care for older people. Recent publications include: W. Tadd & A. Bayer, 'Dignity in health and social care for older Europeans: implications of a European project', *Aging Health* 2 (2006); and G. Woolhead, W. Tadd, A.J. Boix-Ferrer et al., '"Tu" or "vous"? A European qualitative study of dignity and communication with older people in health and social care settings', *Patient Education and Counseling* 61 (2006).

Britt-Marie Ternestedt is professor of nursing and research director at the Department of Palliative Care Research at Ersta Sköndal University College, Stockholm, Sweden. Her research focuses mainly on issues related to death and dying from a life-cycle perspective. She is especially interested in the culture of dying patients and their families and what the parties involved consider to be important values. Two recent articles are: I.L. Källström Karlsson, M. Ehnfors & B.-M. Ternestedt, 'Five nurses' experiences of hospice care in a long-term perspective', *Journal of Hospice and Palliative Nursing* 10 (2008); and E. Ekwall, B.-M. Ternestedt & B. Sorbe, 'Recurrence of ovarian cancer – living in a limbo', *Cancer Nursing*, 30 (2007).

An Outline of the Book

Chapter 1: Basic concepts

In this chapter a number of basic concepts related to health care and the care of older people are analysed. The analysis has a special focus particularly on the notions of health and quality of life. Nordenfelt starts by discussing two notions of health: a biological and scientific notion and an evaluative and holistic one. Nordenfelt opts for using the term 'health' in an evaluative and holistic sense. He characterises health as a person's ability to realise vital goals given standard or otherwise acceptable circumstances. With regard to quality of life, Nordenfelt analyses some arguments in favour of a subjective interpretation. Researchers in the field of medicine and social policy have for a long time used traditional medical and social indicators for measuring both people's health and their welfare. Now they want to know *how people themselves assess their lives*. Nordenfelt argues that there is a call for an assessment of the subject's own evaluation of their state of health or welfare. This means that Nordenfelt in fact equates quality of life with happiness.

The chapter concludes with brief analyses of the related notions of autonomy and integrity. Nordenfelt makes the distinction between two uses of the word 'autonomy'. First, autonomy can be viewed as a theoretical property, i.e. a degree of power and independence, but second it is often viewed as a right. The latter is the case when we claim that a person's autonomy should be respected. What we respect is then the person's right to have and execute a certain power and independence.

Chapter 2: Ideas of dignity

Four types of dignity are distinguished:

- *Human dignity or Menschenwürde* pertains to all human beings to the same extent and cannot be lost as long as the person exists.
- The *dignity of merit* depends on social rank and formal position. There are many species of this kind of dignity and it is very unevenly distributed among human beings. The dignity of merit exists in degrees, and it can come and go.

- The *dignity of moral stature* is the result of the moral deeds of the subject; it can likewise be reduced or lost through the subject's immoral actions. This kind of dignity is tied to the idea of a dignified character and of dignity as a virtue. The dignity of moral stature is a dignity of degree and it is also unevenly distributed among humans.
- The *dignity of identity* is tied to the integrity of the subject's body and mind, and in many instances, although not always, is also dependent on the subject's self-image. This dignity can come and go as a result of the actions of fellow human beings and also as a result of changes in the subject's body and mind.

A person who has a rank or holds an office that entails a set of rights has a special dignity. The dignity of moral stature is a dignity that is dependent upon the thoughts and deeds of the subject. A dignified character is one that is disposed to respect the moral law. The dignity of identity is the dignity that we attach to ourselves as integrated and autonomous persons, persons with a history and persons with a future, with all our relationships to other human beings. Most of us have a basic respect for our own identity, although this identity need not be at all remarkable from a moral or other point of view. But this self-respect can easily be shattered, not only by other human beings but also by nature itself, for instance in the disability of illness and old age.

The German word *Menschenwürde*, usually translated as 'human dignity', refers to a kind of dignity that we as humans all have, or are assumed to have, just because we are humans. This is a specifically human value. We all have this value to the same degree, i.e. we are equal with respect to this kind of dignity. And it is significant that *Menschenwürde* cannot be taken from a human being as long as he or she lives.

Dignity and older people

Is there a dignity particularly attached to older people, which warrants that special attention be paid to them? Or do any of the mentioned varieties of dignity apply more significantly to older people? Nordenfelt argues that *Menschenwürde* is the basic platform. Each older person has his or her intrinsic basic value, which entails a number of rights, among others the rights of the UN Declaration. People do not lose any of these rights because they have reached a particular age. *Menschenwürde* does not, however, cover the whole ground of dignity that is relevant to older people. In this section Nordenfelt discusses whether *wisdom* is a particular dignity that pertains to older people. It is argued that it is a typical virtue of older people to be wise. Hence wisdom might be considered to be a dignity of merit that could be ascribed to older people as a group, although not all individuals among older people exhibit wisdom. Thus, by analogy with *Menschenwürde*, which attaches to all humans regardless of their individual capacities, wisdom can be ascribed to all older people, regardless of their individual abilities and achievements in this respect.

Chapter 3: Being body

In this chapter Jennifer Bullington begins by making clear the distinction between the body-as-thing (third-person perspective) and the body-as-me (first-person perspective).

Owing to the ambiguity of the human body, as embodied consciousness, it is possible to entertain both these notions of the body, even though the body as 'it' or 'thing' is the most common way of conceptualising the body, within both lay and professional language. Over the centuries bodies have been kept out of philosophy, science and other intellectual activities. However, more recently several authors have provided arguments for including the body in the 'higher' functions, such as cognition, imagination and reason.

Following the phenomenologist Maurice Merleau-Ponty, Bullington argues that the subjectivity of the human being is not limited to cases where there is self-consciousness or a specific degree of conscious awareness. A sleeping person is still a subject. A person in a coma is still a subject. Even in sleep or in a coma, the lived body is still 'constituting meaning', although this level of meaning is not the meaning we traditionally refer to when we speak about meaning. The dreamer dreams and the comatose person has experiences. People who have awakened from a coma can relate what they were experiencing during the coma.

Thus, says Bullington, the unconscious person and the demented person too do have a dignity, i.e. the dignity that is implicit in the embodied, first-person point of view. According to phenomenological thinking, this level of dignity must be regarded as primary – that is to say, prior to any conceptualisations of dignity that are based upon psychological traits or social achievements. The dignity of subjectivity has to do with the uniqueness of the lived body and is in a sense another way of describing the universal human dignity of *Menschenwürde*.

Chapter 4: Dignity and dementia

The primary aim of this chapter by Magnus Öhlander is to use ethnographic descriptions of dementia care in a small residential home to analyse the meaning and practice of dignity. How do the staff manage the consequences of dementia and how can this be understood in terms of dignity? How is dignity 'made' in the daily life of the residential home? What can be said from this about the meaning of dignity?

The chapter is empirically based on an eight-month piece of ethnographic fieldwork where participant observation was carried out in a small residential home in Sweden which consists of three merged flats. At the time of the fieldwork six women were living there. The everyday reality of the residential home, the shared world of the women, was a fragile reality. The staff managed this fragile reality in different ways. They could correct 'wrong' interpretations, they could separate the women when they didn't get along and threatened to crack the image of a pleasant time spent together at home, or they could just play along.

Keeping up the 'homelike' framework turned out to be an important ingredient in dignity work. The idea of 'the home' summarises central values, ideals and feelings such as privacy, autonomy, tender care, family, friends, being together, leisure, independence, security, relaxation, cosiness, creativity, the 'I' and the presentation of self. As a symbol, 'home' of course also contains more problematic aspects of life such as gender inequalities, loneliness, isolation, injustice, burdensome childhood memories, violence and assault. In the context of care it is mostly the brighter, more pleasant, positive and salutary aspects that are emphasised.

Chapter 5: Dignity and demented spouses

This chapter by Ingrid Hellström is based on a longitudinal interview study with 20 older people with dementia and their spouses. The aim of the study was to explore the ways in which older people with dementia and their spouses experience dementia over time, especially the impact it has on their interpersonal relationships and patterns of everyday life. Over 150 interviews with the couples were conducted during the period 2001–2006. The interviews with the couples were structured around the themes of the home, memory disturbance, the quality of everyday life and their relationship and dignity and autonomy.

Hellström notes that the aim of sustaining couplehood captured the efforts of both spouses in their interaction. She observes that this involved four interrelated sets of activities: talking things through in order to ensure good communication and acknowledge value differences; being affectionate and appreciative; making the most of things by enjoying everyday pleasures; and finally, keeping the peace by being aware of potential points of friction. Both spouses were active in keeping to this strategy.

Both partners were well aware of the fact that the dementia would get worse over time and this had an influence on their perception of the dignity of the demented spouse. This was salient after some time, especially when communication declined or when the demented spouse was no longer able to live at home.

Chapter 6: Decent care for older people: why dignity matters, the European experience

Win Tadd and Michael Calnan discuss the challenges raised by an ageing population in the Western world, which include a shrinking workforce, pressure on pensions and public finances and an increasing demand for health and social care. These challenges, which affect all European countries to a greater or lesser degree, cannot be met if older people remain the subject of negative stereotyping and discriminatory practices, which detract from their social worth and self-esteem.

Tadd and Calnan point to evidence that suggests that positive health and social outcomes result when people feel more valued and respected, when they are involved in care decisions and are able to exercise direction over their lives. In circumstances where cure is not an option, it seems even more appropriate that care with dignity should become the standard.

This chapter gives an account of the results of the DOE study which explored the experience of dignity from the perspectives of older people, health and social care professionals and young and middle-aged adults in six European countries. In all countries older people emphasised the importance of respect and of receiving recognition from others. The mutuality of respect was frequently mentioned. The second theme was participation and involvement, which were also necessary to experience a sense of dignity. The positive impact on the experience of dignity, deriving from good social relationships, a sense of fulfilment and having a purpose or role in life was discussed in all countries.

The third and largest theme concerned dignity in care, although older participants found it easier to speak of their experiences of indignity than of dignity. They spoke of how they dreaded dependence, of their fear of being a burden and of losing capacity through dementia. Loss of independence was a universal concern.

Chapter 7: Being allowed to be the person one is when close to death

Palliative care concerns optimising the patient's quality of life without shortening or prolonging their existence. Symptom relief is a central component. But that alone is not sufficient, as psychological and existential needs must also be considered. The sick person should also be viewed in his or her social context. This implies that families should be offered support that helps them cope with the difficulties caused by the illness.

Britt-Marie Ternestedt focuses on three perspectives on death. These are usually described as: *traditional death, modern death* and *postmodern death*. They are commonly associated with different periods of societal development. Ternestedt argues that death first changed from a religious event into a medical event. The authority of the clergy and the church was replaced by that of doctors and medical science. As a result, dying, death and the associated rituals became professionalised. The members of the family perceived themselves as being of minor importance, as they were only allowed to visit the patient at fixed times.

Today we have gone a step further. Industrial society has been replaced by an information and knowledge society, where the human being is more or less regarded as an independent actor. If the priest and doctor were previously regarded as authorities, a shift can now be seen towards the individual.

Within palliative care, this means that the dying person is to be regarded as an authority in the sense that he or she is both capable of influencing, and should be allowed to influence, his or her own death. Dying is a unique experience and only the dying person knows deep down what constitutes a dignified death. This person is capable of deciding how to live their final days with the restrictions imposed by the illness. Each individual is unique and has different values and aims in life, which implies that a good death can take many different forms.

Chapter 8: The dignity of the dead

Can a dead person have dignity? Göran Lantz argues for an affirmative answer to this question. He observes among other things the attitude of reverence and awe for a deceased person in funeral practices, evident in all cultures and religions. The idea is often thought to be the strengthening of the bond between the living and the dead. Therefore, the funeral is often associated with a ritual meal, in the Christian tradition

Holy Communion. It is common in certain countries that the gravestone of a person is marked not only with the name of the deceased but also with the title or honours conferred upon them. So it is obviously a fact that people after death may be awarded a dignity of merit, formal or informal. The treatment of the dead according to moral stature can be exemplified by the tradition in the past of burying criminals or people who had committed suicide outside the churchyard or on the north side of the church.

Lantz notes that the idea of a general *Menschenwürde* is primarily applicable to living persons. However, there is a case for attributing dignity and rights to the dead. First, there is a derived or secondary dignity of the dead. That is, the dead person *has been* a human being with full *Menschenwürde*. This fact is mirrored in the dignity and the right to piety that pertains to the dead. Second, we are equal when face to face with death. This goes for both the dying and the dead. An attitude of respect, sympathy and compassion is owed to the dying person. Death is the common end for all living beings. Face to face with death we experience our own mortality and our own anxiety. We share the same fate. And in that sense we are all equal in dignity.

Chapter 9: Experiences from two projects

In this chapter Nordenfelt discusses the problems in research where conceptual analysis encounters empirical studies in which the standard terms for the concepts under scrutiny, such as 'quality of life', 'satisfaction', 'autonomy', 'integrity' and 'dignity', have been used by ordinary native speakers.

The author argues that the purpose of philosophical conceptual analysis is never simply to map ordinary language in all its bewildering variety. The analysis must contain a crucial element of reconstruction and even stipulation. The result of a good conceptual analysis should be a map of a series of concepts that is simpler and more fruitful for further communication than the initial complicated and sometimes even inconsistent map that may be the immediate result of an empirical study.

Finally, the chapter contains a comparison between the results of the two main projects analysed in this book. If one compares the main conclusions of the DOE project with the findings in the Swedish Home project with regard to dignified or good care one can find crucial common themes:

- Supporting and maintaining autonomy, including asking for agreement/consent for the care and letting the power of decision be with the older person (*self-determination*).
- Respecting the patient's home and privacy (integrity) (*self-determination, self-image*).
- Giving personalised support and respecting the individual's habits (*self-image*).
- Giving comfort in living (*synthesis and summation*).
- Not separating or isolating them from life (*social relationships*).
- Giving the necessary care and keeping the person clean (*symptom control*).

Preamble: the Case of David and Rebecca

David was born in northern Norway in 1930. He met Rebecca when he worked as a skiing instructor in the north of Sweden. After a while he moved in with Rebecca, who lived in southern Sweden. David and Rebecca married in 1950 and since 1969 they had lived in a house outside the town, facing on to a forest. They liked their garden and patio very much. They were very active and liked to cycle, go skiing, meet friends, dance – to mention only a few activities. They had one son and two grandchildren who were living in the area and with whom they had a close relationship. David had worked as an engineer. Rebecca had been a housewife and had also worked part-time as a home help.

One day Rebecca was sitting in the living room watching TV when David came in and said, 'I can't count any more'. He told his wife that he had been working the household budget and he was not able to total their monthly bills. Rebecca became worried and then realised that this problem had occurred on earlier occasions. Eventually, David was diagnosed as having Alzheimer's disease. Rebecca remembered that David got his diagnosis on 17 November 2000, and she will never forget that day. They began to adapt to their new situation.

David and Rebecca talked openly about the disease – or rather, she talked openly because her husband sometimes tended to forget he was ill. But when he tried to do things in the house, like cleaning the bathroom, he realised that he was not up to it and became very distressed, and he often cried on these occasions. Rebecca said that she used to hug him and tried to talk about other things. David very much liked to sit beside his wife, holding her hand. He disliked it when she read a book because she was not there for him to the extent he wished. At home, he checked the calendar in the kitchen several times a day to see what day it was and what was planned for the day. Rebecca was his 'memory bank'. She also said that it was important that she should try to remain calm because David was reflecting himself in her. She was like a mirror. When she was upset, he became upset and sad. She knew that she had to rest to be able to support him, and if she needed to rest during the day, her husband sat quietly beside her on the bed and waited for her.

Over time David's memory started to deteriorate and he experienced difficulty in expressing himself. However, the couple were still very active. Rebecca brought her husband along to several activities; however, he did not always know what was happening on these occasions, though his social competence was very much intact, and he appreciated social contacts. The couple were very experienced travellers and had visited several places abroad. They continued to travel after David was diagnosed with Alzheimer's disease, but Rebecca chose destinations that did not put so much pressure on her husband. Bus trips to Germany, for example, worked very well, because he was very pleased when he sat on the bus holding her hand. The last summer they lived in their house, they went on a trip to Norway. Rebecca assumed that this would be their last visit to David's birthplace in northern Norway.

Rebecca did not wish to be called a carer; she was David's wife and she said that since they were married they should help each other. She made plans to leave their house and move to a flat, because she knew that her husband would take up more of her time and she would not be able to cope with a house and garden. From the flat they could easily reach various services like a bus station and shops.

David started to go to a day-care centre three times a week and got on very well. But as time passed his dementia got worse and he went for respite care every fortnight. Rebecca felt that she had let him down because she had set her heart on supporting him to the end. One morning David fell in the bathroom and bumped his head on the washbasin. Rebecca called an ambulance and he was taken to hospital. He recovered from his head injury but unfortunately he got pneumonia and his general health deteriorated rapidly during the following week. Rebecca stayed with him all the time at the hospital. Finally, one evening, David passed away very peacefully with Rebecca and their son at his side.

Reflections

The case of David and Rebecca is a good reflection of what this book is about, i.e. the quality of life and dignity of older people, in particular of those who have lost some of their faculties or whose health has deteriorated. The story of David and Rebecca describes a particularly good case of care. This case is unusual also in the sense that the vulnerable man's carer is his wife.

However, this book also tells stories about bad or even deplorable instances of care – often, significantly enough, in institutions designed for the care of older people. The reasons for the inadequate care vary. Much of course has to do with resources: there is a shortage of staff and lack of utilities. But the explanation also has to do with attitudes and education. Many of the staff looking after older people, even in wealthy European countries, lack adequate training for their job. They have little education and little experience. More importantly, they have had little opportunity to reflect, under good supervision, on the conditions for a high quality of life of their clients and on what constitutes dignified care. One of the main purposes of this book is to provide material for such reflection. It will first offer some conceptual tools. It will ask questions about quality of life and its conditions. It will ask questions about what dignity is, and consider whether there are different kinds of dignity. It will furthermore apply these concepts in various real-life situations, in homes where spouses live together as in the case of David and Rebecca, or in residential homes for older people.

Part I *Theoretical and Conceptual Considerations*

1. *Health, Autonomy and Quality of Life: Some Basic Concepts in the Theory of Health Care and the Care of Older People*

Lennart Nordenfelt

Introduction

In this first chapter a number of basic concepts related to health care and the care of older people are analysed. The analysis focuses particularly on the concepts of quality of life and dignity. These two concepts, however, are not the only ones to be considered in a situation of care. There are other values with which we are perhaps better acquainted and which must play an important role. Among these are health, autonomy and integrity. In this chapter I present some of these values and analyse them to a certain extent. This should make it easier to comprehend the more complicated concepts of quality of life and dignity.

The discussion of quality of life is included in this first chapter since it is so closely related to health, which is the first concept to be studied. The discussion of dignity is held over to the next chapter, where it can be explored in greater detail; this is necessary because the analysis is largely original and some of the ideas are presented here for the first time.

1.1   Health

The most basic of concepts in health care is the concept of health itself. Health is considered by many people, particularly in modern times, to be one of the most precious values in life. They believe that health, and longevity, should be protected and enhanced as much as possible. Thus, the art and science of medicine has received a crucial place in modern society, both Western and Eastern. Doctors are dignitaries. In most countries they are highly regarded and well paid. In some circles they have replaced the priests or even the gods of olden times.

However, one may wonder why health is mentioned in the context of values. Although health is highly regarded it is, one might argue, a state of body or mind that can be scientifically assessed. A doctor or a nurse can investigate a body using modern equipment, taking blood pressure, checking the blood sedimentation rate or using X-ray diagnostics. In such a way health can be exactly determined. This is the view of some experts, in particular some physicians. It is also the view of certain influential philosophers of health.

The most famous protagonist of this view, Christopher Boorse (1977, 1997), defines disease in the following way:

A disease is a type of internal state which is either an impairment of normal functional ability, i.e. a reduction of one or more functional abilities below typical efficiency, or a limitation on functional ability caused by environmental agents.

The notion of functional ability, in this theory, is in turn related to the person's survival and reproduction, i.e. their fitness. The same idea can be formulated in the following positive terms:

A person is completely healthy if, and only if, all their organs function with at least typical efficiency (in relation to survival and reproduction).

However, other experts in the field, both doctors and ethicists, consider that attributing health to a person is not just a matter of scientific investigation. One must also assess how the person feels and what they are able to do in life. It is only when we have knowledge about this *holistic state* of the person that we can attribute health or ill health to them. The healthy person is the person who feels well and can do whatever is needed in their daily life. Moreover, according to this analysis, by designating a state of the whole person as healthy, we have also claimed that this state is a *good* state. Thus we have attributed a value to the person in question. This idea can be developed in at least two directions. Here I will consider, first, health understood as well-being and, second, health understood as a person's ability to realise personal goals.

1.1.1 Health as well-being

It is an important aspect of health that the body and mind are well, in both order and function. But we may ask about the criteria for such well-functioning. How do we know that the body and mind are functioning well? When is the body in balance?

A traditional answer is that the person's subjective well-being is the ultimate criterion (Canguilhem 1978). Simply put: when a person feels well, then they are healthy. This statement certainly entails problems, since a person can feel well and still have a serious disease in its initial stage. The general idea can, however, be modified to cover this case. The individual with a serious disease will sooner or later have negative experiences such as pain, fatigue or mental suffering. Thus the ultimate criterion of a person's health is their present or future well-being. (For a different approach suggesting that complete health is compatible with the existence of disease, see Nordenfelt 1995, 2000.)

It is difficult to characterise the well-being that constitutes health. If we include too much in the concept, there is a risk of identifying health with happiness. Indeed, an accusation commonly directed against the famous WHO definition (1948) is that it falls into this trap. Many critics say that health cannot reasonably be identical with complete physical, mental and social well-being. The absurd conclusion of this conception might be that everyone who is not completely successful in life would be deemed unhealthy.

Some authors (Leder 1990; Gadamer 1993) have pointed out that phenomenological health (or health as it is experienced) tends to remain as a forgotten background. In daily life, health is hardly recognised at all by its subjects. People are reminded of their previous state of health only when it is disrupted – when they experience the pain, nausea or mental suffering of illness. Health is 'felt' only in special circumstances, the obvious example being after periods of illness when the person experiences relief in contrast to their previous suffering.

Thus, although well-being or absence of ill-being is an important trait in health, most modern positive characterisations of health have focused on other traits. One such trait is health as a condition for action, i.e. ability.

1.1.2 Health as ability

A number of authors in modern philosophy of health have emphasised the place of health as a foundation for achievement (Parsons 1972; Whitbeck 1981; Seedhouse 1986; Fulford 1989; Pörn 1993; Nordenfelt 1995). In fact they argue, partly in different ways, that ability/disability is the core dimension determining health or ill health. A healthy person has the ability to perform the actions they need to perform, but an unhealthy person is prevented from performing one or more of these actions. There is a connection between this conception and the one that illness entails suffering. Disability is often the result of feelings such as pain, fatigue or nausea.

The formidable task for these theorists is to characterise the set of actions that a healthy person should be able to perform. Parsons (1972) and Whitbeck (1981) refer to the subject's wants, i.e. the healthy person's being able to do what they want, Seedhouse (1986) to the person's conscious choices, and Fulford (1989) to such actions as could be classified as 'ordinary activities'. I myself settle for what I call the subject's *vital goals*. These goals need not be consciously chosen (babies and people with dementia also have vital goals). They have the status of vital goals because they are states of being that are necessary conditions for the person's happiness in the long run. Health in my theory is thus conceptually related to, but not identical with, happiness. Let me expand on this.

It is plausible to believe that whatever the adequate answer to the question of the nature of health should be, it will be an answer on an abstract level, capable of being summarised in terms of certain general goals. The question to be put should then rather be formulated in the following terms: what are the goals that a healthy person must be able to realise through their actions?

My general proposal (2001, p. 9, slightly revised) is as follows:

A is completely healthy if, and only if, A is in a bodily and mental state which is such that A has at least the second-order ability (i.e. an ability to acquire an ability) to realise all his/her vital goals given a set of standard or otherwise reasonable circumstances.

Let me now clarify and to some extent defend this proposal by commenting on the crucial clauses concerning vital goals and second-order ability. I will be brief with

5

regard to the first clause and instead concentrate on the relation between health and second-order ability.

What are the vital goals of a human being? And is there just one set of vital goals? A person's vital goal, I suggest, is a state of affairs that is necessary for their minimal long-term happiness. As a consequence of this interpretation, many of the things that human beings hope to realise or maintain form part of their vital goals. More precisely, most states that have a high priority on a person's scale of preferences are included in their vital goals. Examples of such vital goals might be passing an exam, or getting married and having children, as well as simply maintaining existing conditions such as retaining one's job and remaining in touch with one's nearest and dearest.

However, certain things that people happen to want do not form part of their vital goals. First, we have trivial wants. We may casually want something, but if we don't get it, it doesn't matter much. Second, people may sometimes have counterproductive wants. They may want to get drunk, but getting drunk is not a vital goal. Instead of contributing to long-term happiness, being drunk contributes in the long run to suffering and thereby unhappiness. Third, we may have irrational wants, i.e. wants that are in conflict with other, more important wants. As soon as someone recognises this conflict, they normally realise that the more important wants are the only candidates for vital goals.

On the other hand, some things that we do not want may be included in our set of vital goals. Completely apathetic or lazy people who do not have any conscious goals whatsoever will soon realise that this creates suffering for them. This will be particularly salient if they do not even seek food or shelter. Getting these basic issues sorted out must certainly form part of long-term minimal happiness, and such basic requirements are among everyone's vital goals.

A crucial observation to be made here, then, is that a vital goal of A need not be wanted by A at a particular moment. A vital goal is thus a technical concept, not identical to the ordinary-language notion of a goal. (For a further discussion, see Nordenfelt 2001.)

I will now turn to the idea of health as a second-order ability. To be healthy, I propose, is to have the second-order ability to realise one's vital goals. Consider the following situation. A refugee from, say, an African country has just moved to Sweden. In his native country he had his own business, which he managed well enough to sustain himself and his family. When he arrives in Sweden he is no longer able to lead such a life. He does not know Swedish culture, particularly the Swedish language, so to begin with he cannot make any arrangements for establishing a business in Sweden. In his home country he lived relatively well, but in Sweden he is disabled. But would we say that this man is healthy in his native country, and becomes ill upon arriving in Sweden? No, it seems more plausible to say that as long as he has the second-order ability to run a business in Sweden, then he remains healthy. This means that as long as the immigrant has the ability to learn the Swedish language and the ability to learn how to cope in Swedish society, then he is a completely healthy person. In general, then, disability that is due solely to lack of training is not an indication of illness. We have reason to speak of illness only if the training process has in turn been prevented by internal factors, in which case there is a second-order disability.

But what about the typical case of illness that is due to an organic disease? Consider the following example. A woman has a first-order ability to perform her professional activities. Then she becomes ill, and as a result loses her first-order ability. But would it be true to say that she no longer has the second-order ability to do her work?

It is easy to be misled here and identify two pairs of concepts that should be kept distinct: one pair is first- and second-order ability, the other is having a basic competence and having the power to execute it. We normally ascribe a basic competence to someone when they know how to do something. According to our previous definition, this need not be true of second-order ability. The immigrant to Sweden has not previously learnt anything about Sweden and does not have the necessary basic competence for making his living in Sweden. He may, however, have the requisite second-order ability.

It is crucial to recognise that a person who has a basic competence vis-à-vis a certain action F need not even have a second-order ability with regard to F. Consider the case of a professional footballer who has broken his leg. Obviously, until he has physically recovered he does not have the first-order ability to play football. Still, we would say that throughout the period of illness he has a basic competence to play football. He knows how to play football. But, while lying in bed or walking on crutches, does he have the second-order ability to play football? No, because having the second-order ability to play football means having the first-order ability to follow a training programme that leads to a first-order ability to play football. But the person who is confined to bed is clearly not in a position to follow such a programme; and so we may say of the footballer that he is ill. The same reasoning may be applied to all paradigm cases of illness due to disease or impairment. During an acute phase of illness, however short it may be, the subject has lost both the first- and second-order ability to perform the actions with respect to which they are disabled.

To this analysis of ability must be added a few remarks about the *circumstances* under which a person can be said to have an ability. It is evident that health cannot be the ability to reach vital goals in all kinds of circumstances. If that were the case then nobody would be completely healthy. There is always some conceivable circumstance in which one cannot reach one's vital goals. The outbreak of a natural catastrophe is one example. Another is that a person may be physically or legally prevented by other people from performing the actions necessary for the achievement of their vital goals. Nor could the ability to realise one's vital goals given just one set of circumstances constitute health. If that were the case, then almost everybody would emerge as completely healthy. Consider the case where an individual is almost completely dependent on the help of someone else in their endeavour to achieve a goal. We can imagine a paraplegic person who is supported in their attempts to reach various destinations; a personal assistant may help in various ways and physically transport the person. If it is true to say that the paraplegic person has the ability to travel wherever they need to go, then we should ascribe health to them. This is clearly counter-intuitive: we do not assess a person as being healthy if they require such extreme support.

So how should these circumstances be defined? One plausible idea is that the circumstances that we normally have in mind in a health assessment are those that are in some way *standard* in our culture. A person who cannot walk on an ordinary pavement is certainly disabled with regard to a standard situation. Likewise, to take an animal example, a dog that cannot run on an ordinary, well-kept lawn is disabled. In both cases, unless there are other impediments, we can draw medical conclusions. The person and the dog are unhealthy.

The way we devise such a standard (which is normally done implicitly) is not via statistics. A situation that is statistically normal in a specific geographical region at a particular time may turn out to be *unreasonable*. In certain countries the political and cultural situation may be such that it is unreasonable to judge the health of its inhabitants given this situation. It may, for instance, be impossible at the moment (January 2009) to work as a teacher in Gaza. But it would be unreasonable to say that the unemployed trained teacher in Gaza is unhealthy for this reason. In this case the circumstances in Gaza are unreasonable.

Although it is evident that health, as ordinarily understood, is connected with ability, and ill health with disability, one may still doubt whether the ability/disability dimension can remain the sole criterion of health/ill health. An important argument concerns those disabled people who are not ill, according to common understanding, and who do not consider themselves to be ill. According to the ability theories of health, these people should be classified as unhealthy.

One answer to this question (Nordenfelt 2001) is that disabled people (given that their disability is assessed in relation to their individual vital goals) are all unhealthy. However, they are not all ill and they do not all have diseases. Another answer, proposed by Fredrik Svenaeus (2001), is that there is a phenomenological difference between the disabled unhealthy person and the disabled healthy person. The unhealthy person has a feeling of not being 'at home' with regard to their present state of body or mind. This feeling is not present for disabled people in general.

I cannot enter further into the difficult discussion about the nature of health here. Suffice it to say that we frequently use the term 'health' in an evaluative sense. When we talk about the desirable state of a human being we may use the terms 'health' and 'healthy'. Health in this sense plays an important role in health care. It defines the goal of care and the framework within which care should be performed. Therefore we can say that health is the basic value in health care.

To summarise: health is the bodily and mental state of a person, often characterised by the person's well-being and, almost universally, by their ability to realise vital goals.

1.2 Quality of life

1.2.1 Introduction

Questions about the relationships between the concepts of health and quality of life have plagued philosophers and empirical researchers in the field of health care for a long time (Nordenfelt 2006). Although much has already been written to clarify the topic, rather little has happened in the field of applications. Much production of instruments is still going on, as if the discussion had not taken place. There is good reason, then, to pursue the philosophical analysis of the topic and also to remind ourselves of the ethical consequences of assessing the quality of people's lives, not least in a situation where this kind of assessment is being made in different ways in different settings and in different parts of the world. In such situations there is hardly any basis for comparing results, but if such a comparison is made notwithstanding, the results can be disastrous.

We can discern three age-old intellectual traditions within which the idea of the good life has been interpreted in quite different ways (Sandöe 1999). The three competing ideas are *perfectionism*, the idea that a person lives a good life when they realise important human potentials; *hedonism*, the idea that a person lives a good life when they seek out certain pleasant states and avoid painful and unpleasant ones; and finally *preferentialism*, the idea that a person lives a good life when they manage to get what they want. These ideas indicate quite different ways of pursuing the good life, and as a consequence the ways by which we can judge the quality of a person's life must be quite different.

But an important question, of course, is why we are investigating the nature of the good life. Perhaps the context can help us in assessing this. As Georg Henrik von Wright pointed out in a classic work (1963), there is a great variety of goodness. The goodness of a good person is different from the goodness of a heart or the goodness of a knife. And a person can be good in several ways: good manners, a good intellect or good sporting ability, for example. It is obvious that there is a multiplicity of dimensions of goodness. But is it reasonable to believe that we can be asking questions about all these dimensions in the discussion about quality of life?

A primary observation is that we must concentrate on a dimension pertaining to human beings. The people who request assessments of quality of life, for instance politicians and researchers in medicine and the social sciences, are asking for the quality of the life of a *human being*. Moreover, the quality should concern the human being as a whole. Still, when we focus on medicine and social affairs the quality of life does not include all aspects of a person (see Nordenfelt 1994). The questions asked within these discourses do not, for instance, concern the moral value of the person in question, nor do they concern aesthetic or intellectual values. It is salient that the concern is rather about what could, at least vaguely, be called the *welfare* of the person. Central in these discourses are questions about how life (in the form of external and internal events) is treating the person. Questions about how the person lives their life, in the sense of how they plan and make choices in life, are less central. Questions like these would of course be particularly pertinent if the discourse concerned moral or intellectual aspects of life.

When one narrows the scope somewhat in this way, it seems that perfectionism is not such a plausible candidate for interpreting the modern notion of quality of life. The traditional, classic version of perfectionism (Aristotle 1934) is indeed an all-encompassing idea about the good life but it has a very strong moral foundation. Moreover, its basic tenet is that *eudaimonia*, the perfect life, consists mainly in the person's virtuous activity.

But even if we focus on welfare we are left with a broad concept, and we can still disagree about what welfare ultimately is. We can wonder whether it has to do primarily with the possession of certain objective properties such as money, a job, freedom from political oppression or freedom from disease, or with an individual's judgement of their situation, or with the presence of certain pleasant mental states in the individual.

Observe that the answer to the conceptual question concerns whether welfare *consists in* certain objective factors, or in such factors as are positively judged by the subject, or in certain pleasant mental states of the subject. Taking a definite stand on this issue does not prevent us from observing the variety of empirical connections between these three ontological categories. One obvious connection is that certain external states of affairs, such as money and a good job, are normally preferred by the subject and normally contribute causally to their pleasure. In such cases there is a congruence in practice between the main theories. A judgement about the presence of high quality of life would be similar from whichever platform we were to judge. But, of course, this need not always be the case.

Much of the present discussion on quality of life in the fields of medicine and social policy focuses on choices between these three theoretical platforms. There seems, however, to be a reasonable consensus that we should not ask for a purely objective measure. We should reconsider the motivation for the introduction of the 'quality of life' concept. The concept was introduced, in medicine, as a supplement to ordinary medical 'objective' judgements of people's health. Doctors and researchers explicitly wanted to know whether the functional improvement of a heart or a lung had really improved the life of the individual. The objective anatomical and functional measure had always been there, but now there was a need for information that went beyond this basic biological knowledge. This new knowledge might still contain certain objective features, but then on the molar level of the person. It might concern abilities such as the ability to walk or use one's hands, but it must also include certain mental features of the person such as preferences, attitudes and emotions.

This argument implies that the shift within medicine to considering the quality of a person's life (from roughly a welfare point of view) means a step away from a biological objectivistic position. Similarly, the concept of 'quality of life' was introduced into social policy as a supplement to the welfare studies in terms of standard of living that had previously been prevalent. A good example of this type of study is the Swedish Annual Surveys of Living Conditions, where facts concerning work, income, housing, education and social mobility are characterised with the help of statistical data (*Living Conditions and Inequality 1975–1995*, Report 91, Statistics Sweden).

One could then ask: What are the reasons for preferring one sense of quality of life to the other? What should our criterion for choice be? Should we make an ordinary-language analysis of the general concept of welfare and examine our intuitions about this concept? Or should we analyse the medical and social contexts in great detail and see what kind of measure is actually being asked for? This method is sometimes preferred (see Birnbacher 1999). For a long time researchers in the field of medicine and social policy used traditional medical and social indicators for measuring people's health and welfare. Now they want to know *how people themselves assess their lives*. Birnbacher asserts, for instance, that there is really a call for an assessment of the subject's own assessment of their state of health or welfare.

If this is in fact the case, the question has been simplified and the theoretical problems have been considerably diminished. In the case where the term 'quality of life' indeed *means*, and should be interpreted as, the subject's assessment of their own situation, then the basic conceptual problem has come much closer to its solution. However, significant problems remain, and they are not just technical. Let me just mention two major problem areas here. The first concerns whether individuals are to be asked to assess their situation in the sense of describing the situation in as neutral a way as possible, or whether they are to evaluate it in normative terms. To put it concretely: is the individual to say, 'I cannot move around as much as I could before', or, 'My present disability makes my life miserable'. It is clear that the same 'objective' disability can mean quite different things to different people. The second major question concerns the question of whether quality of life measures should be partial or total. Should individuals assess their total state of health or total welfare situation, or just certain relevant parts? Can the parts be isolated? Is it reasonable to try to isolate them?

I would argue strongly for adopting a subjectivist and preferentialist interpretation of quality of life, since a subjectively evaluated quality of life is a universal value. Moreover, I would say that a subjectivist concept is largely independent of changing social and cultural values. A further pragmatic reason is that a subjectivist approach is preferable because test *instruments* must ultimately be based on the subject's evaluations. This means, moreover, that these instruments must be individualised to a much greater extent than they normally are now.

An interesting ethical argument for adopting a subjectivist concept of quality of life is also possible. It is clear that the subjectivist approach has anti-paternalistic potential. It is much more in line with respecting the patient as a person to ask how they regard a particular treatment, or how they assess their state of well-being. Indeed, it is difficult to involve patients in decisions about treatment, as the principle of autonomy requires, unless they can first assess their condition.

There is an important set of arguments, then, for adopting a subjectivist and preferentialist notion of quality of life in the contexts of medicine and social policy. Some theoreticians in the field have indeed adopted this notion and have consequently constructed measuring instruments based exclusively on it (see, for instance, 'The General Well-Being Schedule' and 'The Quality of Life Index', McDowell & Newell 1987, pp. 125–133 and 209–213).

It is salient, however, that most instruments, in particular those used for measurement in health care, are much less clear in their conceptual underpinning. They normally contain a substantial element of subjective assessment (in either the hedonistic or the preferential sense). But in addition there are normally elements of an objective kind, for instance in terms of objective symptoms or disabilities (e.g. the modern instrument EuroQuol, Williams 1995). The latter statement can perhaps be countered by noting that it is normally individuals who are asked to make 'objective' assessments about their own symptoms or abilities. On the other hand, these individuals are not normally then asked to evaluate the impact of such a symptom or disability. One may wonder what the constructors of such instruments think they are doing. Do they believe that it is not necessary to be clear about the basic concept? Or do they think that there is a merit in mixing concepts in one and the same instrument?

For my present purposes I will adopt a subjectivist notion of quality of life which I call *happiness with life*.

1.2.2 The concept of happiness
My basic intuition concerning happiness is the following:

> Sara is happy with her life as a whole if, and only if, Sara wants her life-conditions to be exactly as she finds them to be.

A way of expressing this intuition is to say that there is an equilibrium between Sara's wants and reality as she finds it. I call this notion *happiness as equilibrium*. It follows from this characterisation that happiness must be a dimensional concept. Sara is more or less happy with life according to the degree of agreement between the state of the world as she sees it and her wants. Moreover, she can be completely happy with life only if her life-conditions are exactly as she wants them to be. Similarly, she is completely unhappy with life only if nothing in her life is as she wants it to be. There is, then, a continuum from complete happiness to complete unhappiness. This continuum must be distinguished from any particular state of happiness.

The opposition between happiness and unhappiness is of a contradictory kind. This means that the continuum can be divided into two mutually exclusive parts: one part of happiness and another part of unhappiness. Later I shall try to characterise the point at which happiness and unhappiness meet. I shall suggest a notion of minimal happiness based on the concept of a high-priority want.

To the global notion of happiness with life corresponds a molecular notion of happiness with a particular fact. Sara can, for instance, be happy with the fact that she has passed an exam. She is happy because she wanted to pass this exam. In general, Sara is happy with every fact that constitutes the satisfaction of a want of hers. In a way global happiness with life constitutes the sum of molecular happiness with particular facts. The sum, however, cannot be derived in a simple arithmetical way.

Our general happiness or unhappiness concerning life is dependent, not so much on the number of things that we are happy about, but on what kinds of things we are happy about, in particular on what we consider to be important in life. To most of us it is more important to become a parent than to have a nice day out in the countryside. A father's happiness about his newborn baby influences his general happiness much more than his happiness about the beautiful weather. I shall return to this in a more systematic way later on.

1.2.3   The reference of happiness to different points in time
I said that Sara is happy now if the state of the world is as she wishes it to be. This reference to the present is important and requires further comment. It is plausible to think in the following way: if happiness is connected with the fact that wants have been satisfied, then happiness ought to be connected with the past. That person is happy, one might think, whose wants in the past, including the most recent past, have been realised. I can easily show that this idea is not sufficient to explain the nature of happiness. Consider the following case:

> A small boy has wanted for a long time to have an electric train. He has wanted this intensely and told his parents about his desire. He is given this toy train as a Christmas present. He certainly becomes very happy. However, after a short while he becomes terribly bored. He finds that there is in fact very little that he can do with the toy. His happiness has very quickly been transformed into boredom.

What has happened, if we wish to describe this situation in more abstract terms? It is true that the boy has had a want from the past satisfied. However, this want no longer exists. At the present moment there is no want for the train; therefore the presence of the train cannot satisfy a want on the part of the boy; therefore it cannot contribute to his happiness.

The important and indeed well-known lesson to be learnt from this example is that the satisfaction of wants can be followed by emotions such as disappointment, boredom and regret. Therefore the wants whose satisfaction should constitute happiness must refer to the present. The reference to the present solves a further problem that is often mentioned in dissertations about happiness. A person can say, 'I am happy about the gift that I have received, but I had never expected to receive it and I had never wanted it.' It can very well happen that something new occurs in one's life and one may not even have known of its existence; therefore one cannot have wanted it in the past. But when it occurs, one may quite strongly want to hold on to it – one likes it, as we say. Thus its existence at the present time contributes to one's happiness.

But what about wants which are directed towards the distant future? Do they have anything to do with one's happiness? Consider a young man who is planning his life. He intends to marry in ten years, he plans to complete an education that takes at least five years, and after that he wishes to enter upon a long career as, say, a lawyer. In short, he has many wants referring to the very distant future. By definition, these wants cannot be satisfied now. If they could, they would not be wants directed towards the future. But what does that mean for the happiness of the young man? Is he extremely unhappy? A moment's reflection shows that this would be an absurd conclusion.

Again, this case shows that happiness is dependent on those wants that refer to the present. And indeed, wants that are directed towards the future sometimes have important implications for the present. In order to take one's law degree in five years' time it may be necessary to begin the relevant education right away. Therefore this future-directed want implies a present-directed want and if this present-directed want is not satisfied now, then the person has reason to be unhappy.

1.2.4 The dependence of happiness on belief and knowledge
In order to be able to want something, one must be a minimally intellectual creature. One cannot want to have a car unless one can imagine a car. One cannot want to take an exam if one does not know anything about exams and their relevance for certain professional careers.

This truth has immediate consequences for the concept of happiness that I am attempting to establish. I cannot be happy about a gift unless, at least, I believe that I have received this gift. The sources of this belief, however, can be of various kinds and various validities. Most importantly, they can be either true or false.

If John is happy about an event, then John believes (or knows) that this event has occurred and that this constitutes the satisfaction of a want of his. But as I said before, this belief need not agree with reality; what it agrees with is John's perception and awareness of reality.

John may have good reasons for his beliefs. He may have observed the occurrence of the event in question, or he may have perfectly trustworthy informants. In such a case we could say that John's happiness is rationally founded. Some authors require such a rational foundation in order for the happiness to be a real human good or to be considered to constitute a high degree of quality of life. The Swedish philosopher Bengt Brülde (1998, 2007) argues strongly for the requirement of rationality. It proves, however, to be quite difficult to spell out exactly what this requirement involves. See Egonsson (2006) for a thorough analysis of this problem.

The concept of happiness to be established is thus cognitive. This leads us to a reflection on other positive, non-cognitive, states of mind. What is the relation of each to happiness?

1.2.5 On happiness and pleasure

What is the relation between pleasure and happiness? Let me try to answer this question by considering what can be a reason for wanting something. Why do we want to have something – why, in general, do we want something to be the case? We can give many answers to such 'why' questions, and they can be different for different people. But there is a typical answer to such questions: I want x because x gives me immediate pleasure. This is a way of terminating the series of 'why' questions. There is no point in asking further questions.

There is a famous theory called *psychological hedonism* which states something as strong as the following: all our wants refer ultimately to a state of pleasure of some kind. The pleasure need not be the immediate reason; the chain often has more than one link. It can have the following structure:

I want to have a car at hand to be able to get to the theatre.
I want to get to the theatre to see an interesting play.
I want to see this play for the sake of intellectual pleasure.

This hierarchy of wants that terminates with the want for pleasure is indeed typical. I do not, however, as the psychological hedonists do, consider it to be the only kind of hierarchy that there is.

Pleasures are states of mind that are typically wanted for their own sake. This does not, however, mean that pleasure is identical with happiness, nor that a person who experiences strong pleasure is automatically happy. A person is of course normally happy about pleasure, or about the absence of pain, but there are cases where this need not be so. Consider the case where the pleasure is a sign that something dangerous is going on – the pleasure involved in taking a drug, for instance. The addict may be conscious of the fact that after a while the pleasure will be gone and the future suffering will be great. Hence, although at a particular moment the addict may experience intense pleasure, they may at the same time be deeply unhappy.

Conversely, pain and suffering are states of mind that are typically unwanted. Normally, a person in great pain is unhappy about their state of mind. But again this need not be so. The pain or suffering may be a sign that something positive is coming. For example, a surgical operation may be quite painful. However, if the patient believes that the operation is an effective measure and that they will soon be healthy, then the pain is easily endurable and can coexist with great happiness.

1.2.6 On different degrees of happiness

I have said that happiness can be viewed as a dimension. A person can be more or less happy. But how should we understand this dimension? And what determines a person's degree of happiness?

Since happiness is conceptually connected to the agreement or disagreement between a person's wants and reality as they find it, it is tempting to relate happiness to the number of wants that have been realised. Suppose that John has 100 wants and that 90 of them have materialised. Suppose, on the other hand, that Sara has as many wants but that only 10 of them are realised. According to a simple arithmetical calculation, John's happiness ought to be 9/10 of the possible total happiness, whereas Sara only reaches 1/10 of total happiness. Hence John must be much happier than Sara.

A moment's reflection shows that this reasoning must be a caricature, for a number of reasons. One important reason has to do with the idea of a want-unit. What is *one* want as opposed to a number of wants? Is my want now to scratch my nose to be compared to my want to protect my family from harm? And what about a hierarchy of wants? Consider the case of going to the theatre presented above. Are we talking there about three wants or just about one basic want?

I have said enough to introduce some major problems, but I shall not go deeper into them now. It is not necessary for my main reasoning, which will completely avoid the counting of wants. Instead, I shall introduce the idea that there are wants of higher and lower *priority*. It is the degree of priority that determines whether or not great happiness will result from the satisfaction of a want.

Some of our wants are of vital importance to us. To most of us it is very important that our family should be well and successful. Our own health is also of great importance. So is the fact that our professional situation is all right, and perhaps also that the political situation is tolerable. The fact that these conditions hold has considerably higher priority than most other things we wish to do or have at a particular moment.

Thus there must be a scale of priority or importance along which we can rank our wants. This ranking is practically never explicit, nor is it particularly clear when we try to visualise it. Certainly there is no 'naturally' given cardinal order for these wants. We cannot say that it is five times more important that our children are alive than that our own health is in order. But what, then, can we say about this scale of priority that certainly exists in every human being? First, how can we know that a certain want of Sara's has a higher priority than another, or what the criterion for this is? I suggest the following characterisation:

Sara's want to have *x* has a higher priority for her than Sara's want to have *y* if, and only if, in a choice between *x* and *y*, where both cannot be realised, Sara would prefer *x*.

With this formulation I can keep the connection to my basic analysis of the concept of happiness. I said that Sara is happy about life if, and only if, Sara wants the conditions of life to be exactly as she finds them to be. We can now say that Sara is happier about a situation *x* than about another situation *y* and explain it by simply saying that Sara prefers *x* to *y*.

Given this explication, we seem to have an intrapersonal instrument for comparison. We can understand how to analyse and also in principle how to get to know that an individual is happier now than they were before. But do we now have an instrument for a comparison between different people? How shall we explicate the idea that Smith is happier than Brown, or for that matter that Smith and Brown are equally happy? The analysis given above will allow us to do this only under very specific circumstances. Assume that Smith and Brown have exactly the same profile of wants. That is, they have exactly the same wants and their priorities among the wants are identical. Thus

15

we know that, if Smith prefers x, Brown must also do so (given that x and y are total situations). Assume now that Smith is in a situation x and Brown is in y. Then it follows that Smith is happier than Brown.

A pragmatic method for interpersonal comparison of happiness would then be to describe their respective life situations to the people involved. To make it as simple as possible: we compare the happiness of two people, John and Sara. We describe John's situation meticulously to Sara, and vice versa. It appears that John prefers his own situation to Sara's and that Sara prefers John's situation to her own. Then we have reason to say that John is happier than Sara.

Having described this procedure for interpersonal comparison, I must point out two great difficulties in practice. 'Preference' in this context is an ideal concept. We must be talking about an ideal situation of choice, where the individual has complete self-knowledge and can foresee such things as risk of disappointment or boredom. It is certainly true that people normally lack this self-knowledge in actual situations of choice. It is also important to stress that one has to compare people's total situations in order to be sure that the result mirrors their states of happiness. Smith who is in situation x need not be happier than Brown who is in y (even if both of them prefer x to y) if x and y do not cover total life situations. If x and y only affect some part of their lives, for instance professional life and state of health, then it is always possible that something unhappy has occurred to Smith in some other sphere of his life. He may have lost some close relative, which has caused him deep grief.

In general it is easy to go wrong when one dreams about another person's life situation and prefers it to one's own. It was easy to prefer the life of Aristotle Onassis to one's own. But one must remember that his life-situation consisted not only of his money and his yachts but also his poor health and his love problems.

How, then, should we treat all those cases where people's goal profiles differ and where a comparison between the life situations of two people does not result in both agreeing on which situation to prefer? Can we then ever say that one person is happier than another?

My general conclusion is that there are many cases where the happiness of one person and that of another are incommensurable. In these cases – for theoretical as well as practical reasons – we simply cannot say that one person is happier than the other. There is one important exception to this, however. This is the case where John finds his situation unacceptable, while Sara finds hers acceptable. In this case Sara is clearly happier than John. And we can say this even if Sara were to prefer John's situation to her own, and John were to prefer his to Sara's.

The notion of *acceptability* indicates where the line is between happiness and unhappiness on the happiness scale. For every human being there is a level that marks the transition from happiness to unhappiness. Below this level the situation is so far from satisfactory that it is not acceptable to the individual. They are unhappy. Just above this level the situation is acceptable; they are minimally happy.

We can make a preliminary characterisation of this line in the following way: in order for John to be at least minimally happy, then all those conditions that have a high priority for John, in an absolute sense of the word, must have materialised.

Where this line goes in any concrete sense must vary greatly between different people. People have different temperaments and character traits. Impatient or spoilt people become unhappy for the most trivial reasons. For such people almost every want has a high priority. Patient or stoic people, on the other hand, can meet most adversities without falling below the 'acceptable' level. To such people very few things in life have a high priority.

This observation about the dependence of happiness on how we set our priorities contains a key to happiness which I have hitherto not recognised. To influence a person's happiness means not only to try to realise states of affairs in their external or internal situation. It equally entails influencing their profile of wants. The person who has a low profile, the person with the smallest number of high-priority wants, has, in one sense, the greatest chance of becoming happy.

1.2.7   On the relation between health and quality of life

I suggest here an interpretation of quality of life such that there is a clear distinction between health and quality of life. In fact, it is only if we can find a substantial difference between them that we need both concepts.

It is easy to see that health and quality of life are different when we consider that quality of life may involve matters external to the individual. A person is said to have a high quality of life if they possess great wealth or have good opportunities to travel and have a great variety of experiences. Health does not have to do with such external facts.

In another usage of the term, which I think is the basic one, quality of life refers to a person's degree of happiness. An extremely happy person has a high quality of life; an unhappy person has a low quality of life. We can distinguish health from quality of life in this usage too. A healthy person need not be happy. Consider the healthy man who has just lost one of his children. This man is extremely unhappy as a result, but his health may very well remain intact. Conversely, consider an old woman who is dying and does not have many more days to live. She may be dying in a peaceful way; she may have her family with her all the time and may be pleased with the fact that she has lived a long and successful life. She may be very ill, but at the same time quite happy.

Thus health is different from quality of life, but the two are related. It is significant that health *normally* contributes to a high quality of life and that ill health *normally* contributes to a low quality of life. The value of health is therefore connected to the value of quality of life.

We can say that quality of life is a value that lies beyond health. In health care, for instance, we may contribute to a person's quality of life *by* enhancing their health. This is a typical way of improving quality of life, but it is not the only way. Quality of life can be enhanced more directly. A dying person may be in great pain, and such pain can be suppressed by pain-killing drugs. As a result the quality of life of the person, but hardly their health, will be enhanced. Many acts of care, however, do not directly involve the physical treatment of a body. They may be acts of charity and kindness, or acts of encouragement and consolation. Such acts can moderate a patient's unhappiness and increase their level of happiness.

Therefore quality of life, in the sense of happiness, can also be a direct goal of health care. (See also in this context the Final Report of the Swedish Parliamentary Priorities Commission: *Priorities in Health Care: Ethics, Economy, Implementation*, Government

Official Reports 1995:5, where quality of life is given the status of a goal of medicine alongside the traditional goal of health.) This does not mean that all kinds of enhancement of happiness are proper parts of health care. Intervention in a person's financial situation falls outside its remit; so does intervention in their love life.

Quality of life in the happiness sense seems to be closely related to the satisfaction of the person's deepest wants. To put it simply: a person is happy with life when their deepest wants are satisfied or there is a good prospect that they will be satisfied.

1.3 Autonomy

1.3.1 Introduction

Autonomy derives from two Greek words, *auto* meaning self and *nomos* meaning rule or law. Literally, then, autonomy has to do with setting rules for oneself. This literal sense is also the basic one adopted by the philosopher Immanuel Kant (1724–1804); see Kant (1997). To him, the autonomy of the human being is one of the most characteristic properties of humanity. Human beings, in contradistinction to animals, have autonomy, entailing the power to set rules for themselves. They create their own ethics and legal systems. 'Autonomy indicates the ability of the human being to be a self-legislative rational being, having the capacity to recognise the universal validity of moral law without being determined by outer heteronomous conditions for action' (Rendtorff & Kemp 2000, p. 26).

In modern medical ethics a much wider concept of autonomy has emerged. Autonomy in this sense concerns individuals' general ability to handle their own affairs, in particular their ability and opportunity to decide for themselves. Thus autonomy has become a general concept of power, freedom and independence. 'For many people today, moral autonomy is a question of free moral choice according to a set of values that the individual finds right and just. And to be morally autonomous is related to sincere choice and personal decision-making' (Rendtorff & Kemp 2000, p. 27).

Some recent studies in medical ethics have emphasised that the moral choice need not be individual. In many instances, both in health care and in ordinary life, decision-making is shared between two or more people. Zeiler (2005) gives a detailed analysis of the case where a couple together make the crucial decision of having pre-implantation genetic screening and possibly having a fertilised egg implanted in the woman's uterus. Here Zeiler emphasises that the decision is shared and the question of whether such a choice is autonomous or not concerns the couple as a unit and not the individuals separately. The issue of couplehood is also raised in the context of the Home project. Hellström (2005) describes how a couple where one of the spouses is demented share much of the decision-making and act together. For details of this study, see Chapter 5 of this book.

We commonly say that we have a duty to respect a person's autonomy. (For the sake of simplicity, in the following I will stay with the case of individual decision and action.) This is shorthand for saying that we must respect a person's *right* to autonomy. What we mean then is that we must respect every individual's right to decide for themself. This is central in the setting of medical care and the care of older people. Everyone has in principle the right to decide with regard to their own affairs. Everyone has the right to choose what to wear, how to spend their days, where to travel, and so on. All patients also have crucial rights with regard to their treatment and care. In particular, they have the right to refuse treatment and care. In principle, no treatment or care can be forced upon anyone. This rule is included in the health-care legislation of many Western countries, although there are, however, justified exceptions to this rule dealing with the care and treatment of babies and of people with dementia or psychosis.

Autonomy, in the sense of ability and opportunity for decision, has gradually become an extremely important value in medicine and care in general. There is perhaps a special emphasis on this value at the present time. Up to the Second World War, medical treatment and care almost totally lacked respect for patient autonomy. We can say that the system of health care in those days was *paternalistic*.

1.3.2 Paternalism and autonomy

Consider now the following slightly paradoxical dictum that can be heard defended in contemporary medical and social ethics (cf. for instance Seedhouse 1991, pp. 113–119):

> It is sometimes right to violate a person's autonomy in order to increase his or her future autonomy.

What does this mean? Is it indeed a paradox? And does the word 'autonomy' mean the same thing both times it is used? To illustrate this, consider the usual situation in schools, where the teachers have quite a paternalistic attitude towards their students. The latter are always being told by their teachers what to do and what to study. In spite of some recent changes, the students have rather little to say about how their education should be planned and carried out. This situation prevails for quite a long period of children's lives. Thus we can say that for rather a long time they have little autonomy. Perhaps we might even say that their autonomy is being violated during this period. On the other hand, this type of paternalistic education is normally defended. Most of us would argue that the intention behind traditional school education is benevolent. Some people would even say that the institution of the school is working for the autonomy of the pupils in the long run. The school is designed to prepare the children to become autonomous adults.

It is easy to construct similar examples from medical ethics. The doctor, or the health-care worker in general, may enforce a certain treatment on a particular patient, and thereby violate the patient's autonomy, but does so in the name of this patient's future autonomy. Without the treatment, the health worker says, the patient will, for instance, not be able to form autonomous decisions in the future.

I think we understand the reasoning here quite well. Especially in our role as parents, we are all too familiar with it. But there are a number of puzzling theoretical issues that need clarification here. Perhaps the most important question is the following: Is the autonomy that we say is being violated the same thing as the autonomy of the future autonomous agent? My main task in the present section is to discuss this problem.

First, we need to make the well-known distinction between autonomy as a theoretical property and autonomy as a normative property. Or, to put it more clearly: we should distinguish between, on the one hand, a person's property and, on the other hand, their right to have this property.

When we violate a pupil's or patient's autonomy, strictly speaking we violate their right to have or execute this autonomy. On the other hand, when we raise the level of a person's autonomy, we do not, at least not in the examples cited, increase this person's right to autonomy but rather we increase the amount to which some theoretical property is instanced in the person.

Of course, we can also conceive of a case of raising or enforcing the right to autonomy, for instance when we campaign politically for patients' rights, or when, as legislators, we actually enforce the rights of certain groups of people. But in our example this is not the case. When we educate or cure people and claim that we thus raise the level of their autonomy, we are not raising the level of their political rights. Instead, we are trying to raise the level of some theoretical property of the people in question.

But what is this property? And are we talking about the same property in the first use of the word as in the second? Do we have the right to autonomy in the same sense as when we say that we wish to see somebody's autonomy increased? These are my principal questions.

Let me analyse this stepwise. Consider first what is being violated in the medical ethics case. Assume that some health-care officials initiate an inoculation programme without consulting any members of the community, or even their political representatives. We then accuse the officials of violating the people's autonomy. What do we mean? In what sense has the autonomy of the members of the community been violated?

The obvious answer is that the health officials have violated the people's right to decide about their own situation. They have prevented them from making an autonomous decision in this particular case of disease prevention. There may even be two elements in this violation of the people's rights. First, there is a lack of information about the planned measures; second, there is an attempt to force the people to comply with these measures.

There are then two rather specific rights that are violated: the right to be informed about a matter of vital concern to oneself and the right to decide concerning this matter. The violation entails that these rights are prevented from being executed in this situation. The violation does not, however, affect the existence of the rights. In fact, in order to be able to talk about a violation of a right we must presuppose the existence of this right.

Let me now turn to an analysis of the theoretical property of autonomy. What is it to be an autonomous agent? The etymological basis is of importance here, as emphasised by Dworkin (1976) among others. 'Autonomy' means self-government. The autonomous person can govern their own life. This can have a number of implications, of which the most important seem to be that the autonomous person makes their own decisions, not forced by any other person. Moreover, the autonomous person acts according to these decisions. No other person prevents them from executing the decisions. This is a minimal definition of autonomy as freedom to decide and act.

So far I have only discussed freedom in so-called interactional terms, i.e. in terms of freedom from human intervention. The concept can, however, be generalised to cover freedom from all kinds of intervention. The autonomous person is then not forced by any external force whatsoever, be it human or non-human. Examples of non-human forces are acts performed by other living beings, such as apes or dogs, and by natural forces such as hurricanes and earthquakes.

Now we have a slightly broader notion of autonomy as freedom from external intervention in deciding and acting. It is likely that autonomy as a right is normally seen to be connected to this sense. This right would reasonably exclude most instances of human interaction of the coercive kind. It is doubtful, however, whether it should also cover most non-human interaction. I think that the right extends only to such non-human interference as could reasonably be prevented by human measures. Certain natural catastrophes would presumably fall outside the framework.

A full philosophical analysis of this kind of freedom requires more. Dworkin, who has contributed much to this analysis, notes that freedom from interference must not entail that one could not be influenced by other agents. The autonomy that we wish to establish in the context of rights must be compatible with receiving information and even recommendations from other agents. The important feature is that we, as agents, should be able to evaluate the information and recommendations in the light of our basic values.

Freedom from external interference, however, need not be the whole story. In order to be an autonomous agent in the full-blown sense of the word one must not be disturbed by internal interference either. By this I mean interference from intoxication by alcohol or drugs, or indeed the abstinence from such substances. A person who is in a state of abstinence and craves more drugs does not, we would say, have the free will to act. The agent in such a case does not have the opportunity for free deliberation. The urge for the drugs and thereby for a continuation of the self-destructive life is too strong.

But from here it is not a big step to the kind of internal interference that is constituted by mental illness. Someone with severe schizophrenia may be unable to reflect upon their situation and weigh alternatives in the light of their deepest values. Mental illness can disable a person with regard to decision-making capacity as well as capacity for action. But mental illness is only the most radical compromiser of autonomy: it is a typical feature of all kinds of diseases that they compromise ability in some way. When one is ill, one is typically unable to do what one wants to do. In fact, one is prevented from realising one's intentions. One's freedom to act is gone. Hence one's autonomy in this extended sense is compromised.

1.3.3 Two notions of autonomy

At this stage of the argument we are not far from identifying the notion of autonomy with the notion of power to act or indeed with the notion of health (in the holistic sense of the word) that some theorists today propose. According to one such notion, which I endorse and have presented more fully above, a person is in complete health if, and only if, given standard or otherwise accepted circumstances, they can realise all their vital goals.

This extended interpretation of autonomy is not far-fetched. David Seedhouse (1988, pp. 132–133) uses the expression 'creating autonomy'. Here he identifies the work for health with the creation of autonomy. The discussion is elaborated in Seedhouse (1991).

But now the central questions of this discussion need to be raised again. The first question relates directly to my initial statement that it is sometimes right to violate a person's autonomy in order to raise the level of their future autonomy. I asked: Do we mean the same by 'autonomy' in the two uses of the word here? The second question is: If we do not mean the same, would it make sense to make a similar claim with an identical meaning in the two uses of 'autonomy'?

As I said, I think that it is relatively easy to identify the ordinary meaning of 'respecting a person's right to autonomy' in the context of medical ethics. The sense normally is: respect this person's right to decide about the measures which are being proposed in order to contribute to their health.

What can we mean, then, when we say that we create autonomy? This is much less clear unless we make some stipulations. One way of interpreting the term is to confine its use to the area of decision-making. In the school situation we may, for instance, justify our paternalism by saying that our education system makes the children much better equipped in the future to make decisions independently of other people. Another, rather extreme, interpretation would encompass the agent's general ability to perform actions. This is the sense partly referred to by Seedhouse in the work cited above. 'The idea of autonomy makes full sense only when it is thought of in terms of being able to do in the widest sense' (Seedhouse 1991). Creating autonomy, according to this interpretation, is partly tantamount to raising the level of a person's general health in a holistic sense of the word 'health' (see my analysis of health above). Observe, however, that autonomy here entails more. Autonomy does not only entail the person's internal *ability* to act, it also entails the person's *opportunity* to act.

An obvious conclusion to be drawn from this analysis is that there must be a difference between the two uses of the word 'autonomy'. Even if the creation of autonomy refers only to the person's ability to make independent decisions, there could be a difference. To respect autonomy in a particular case may concern something very limited, i.e. a right to decide on a particular matter. The creation of autonomy, on the other hand, concerns a *general* ability to make certain kinds of decisions.

A further observation is that when we respect a person's right to decide on a particular matter, we primarily see to it that we ourselves, as external agents, do not prevent the person from forming a decision of their own. Contributing to the creation of a person's autonomy, on the other hand, normally only deals with the strengthening of the person's internal ability to form decisions. The creation of autonomy can hardly include possible future interference in the decision-making on the part of external agents. We can hardly, by any measures that we take today, prevent the appearance of paternalistic officials or doctors in the future. Thus in a sense there is no such thing as creating complete autonomy for the future.

Initially, I also asked the following question. Would it make sense to say: respect a person's right to autonomy in the full-blown sense of autonomy? To elaborate, could we sensibly say: respect a person's right to have the power to work, love and play? And what does it entail? Does such respect, for instance, entail active help and active support from us in the execution of such a power? I merely raise these questions here: a detailed answer would require space that goes beyond the scope of this chapter.

Let me now summarise. A person's 'right to autonomy' in the standard context of medical ethics refers to a person's right to make decisions of their own without being forced by some external agent or some non-human circumstance that could reasonably be prevented by external agents, concerning a health-care or health-promotive measure. It is easy to apply this principle *mutatis mutandis* to the care of older people.

The idea of creating autonomy, on the other hand, which is now being introduced in medical philosophy, refers to the creation of a general ability (and the corresponding opportunity) on the part of the subject, an ability which includes the ability to make

Table 1.1 The various senses of autonomy

Autonomy as a theoretical property	Autonomy as a right
Ability and opportunity to make an informed decision	The right to make an informed decision
General ability and freedom to execute this general ability	The right to execute and develop a general ability in a permissive and supportive environment

independent decisions but which may also include the ability to work, play and love.

The various senses of autonomy analysed in this section can be summarised as a matrix (Table 1.1).

1.4 Integrity

Let me also briefly introduce a further value, integrity, which has a prominent place in health care and the care of older people. This value is closely related to autonomy and can be analysed as a special case of autonomy. The word *integrity* is derived from the Latin *integer*, which means 'whole' or 'undamaged'. To violate the integrity of a person is to violate the wholeness of this person, i.e. it entails hurting them.

There is a value, then, attached to the person's wholeness or identity (a concept that I will return to). This identity can be violated in many ways, some of which have been discussed with regard to health care. The most obvious infringement is the physical one, for instance when the person is intentionally assaulted and hurt. But there are many other possibilities. A person can be debased by improper treatment, for instance by being left naked in front of strangers or being verbally insulted.

Moreover, the person's private arena can be intruded upon. We think that everybody has a right to privacy and that it is an infringement to enter the private arena without permission. This right is particularly obvious when we are talking about the person's property. We cannot enter a person's home without permission and we cannot just seize any of their belongings. But this is not the whole story. Privacy is also a more general concept. We think that everybody has a right to some privacy even in a hospital or a residential home. Although patients may only be allotted a very limited physical space, such as a bed and a bedside table, which they do not own in a legal sense, they can claim a moral right to this space. Any intrusion into this space is a violation unless the patient gives consent or in an emergency situation.

There is a further aspect of integrity that is of particular importance in health care and the care of older people. Much information about people belongs to their private sphere. Doctors and nurses get to know a lot about their patients, including intimate information. This information does not deal only with the physical and mental condition of the patient: it may also concern social circumstances, such as family relationships and the work situation. This is information that people often wish to keep confidential, and revealing it is a serious infringement of their integrity. It is significant that the rule

23

about confidentiality is one of the oldest in the history of medical ethics: it already exists in the ancient Hippocratic oath dating perhaps from the fourth century BC.

The concept of integrity can be widened further to include the individual's life story and life context. Respect for integrity can thus be understood as 'respect for the unity of a life story, a life-context and a life-totality by which we recognise the identity of the other' (Rendtorff & Kemp 2000, p. 39) (see my discussion of dignity of identity, Chapter 2, section 2.2).

1.5   Final remarks on the basic values

How are the values discussed here related to each other? I have already noted the salient relation between health and happiness. Health is causally contributory to a high degree of happiness, but it is neither a necessary nor a sufficient cause of a high degree of happiness. Are there any similar connections between integrity and autonomy on the one hand and quality of life on the other? There are relationships, but they are partly different from the case of health. With integrity and autonomy the most obvious relationship is that somebody respects the integrity and autonomy of the subject in question and the subject's quality of life is enhanced as a result of the respect shown. In the case of autonomy understood as capacity and freedom almost on a par with health, there is a further relationship to note. The person who feels that they are capable and free may be content with the situation and thus have an enhanced quality of life. For a confirmation of such relationships, consider some of the empirical results in Chapter 9.

The relation between integrity and autonomy is salient. Respecting a person's integrity can be looked upon as a special case of respecting autonomy. To respect a person's integrity is at least partially to respect that person's right to decide about their private affairs, including their private space.

References

Aristotle (1934) *The Nicomachean Ethics*. Loeb Classical Library, Harvard University Press, Cambridge, MA.

Birnbacher, D. (1999) Quality of life – evaluation or description. *Ethical Theory and Moral Practice*, **2**, 25–36.

Boorse, C. (1977) Health as a theoretical concept. *Philosophy of Science*, **44**, 542–573.

Boorse, C. (1997) A rebuttal on health. In: *What is Disease? Biomedical Ethics Reviews* (ed. J. Humber & R. Almeder). Humana Press, Totowa, NJ.

Brülde, B. (1998) *The Human Good*. Acta Philosophica Gothoburgiensa 6, Gothenburg.

Brülde, B. (2007) *Lycka och lidande: Begrepp, metod och förklaring* [Happiness and suffering: Concepts, methods and explications]. Studentlitteratur, Lund.

Canguilhem, G. (1978) *On the Normal and the Pathological*. Reidel, Dordrecht.

Dworkin, G. (1976) Autonomy and behavior control. *Hastings Center Report*, **6**, 23–28.

Egonsson, D. (2006) *Preference and Information*. Ashgate, Aldershot.

Fulford, K.W.M. (1989) *Moral Theory and Medical Practice*. Cambridge University Press, Cambridge.

Gadamer, H.-G. (1996) *The Enigma of Health: The Art of Healing in a Scientific Age*. Stanford University Press, Stanford.

Hellström, I. (2005) *Exploring 'Couplehood' in Dementia: A Constructivist Grounded Theory Study*. Linköping University Medical Dissertations No. 895, Linköping.

Kant, I. (1997) *Foundations of the Metaphysics of Morals*. Translated with an introduction by L.W. Beck, Prentice Hall, Upper Saddle River, NY.

Leder, D. (1990) Clinical interpretation: the hermeneutics of medicine. *Theoretical Medicine*, **11**, 9–24.

Living Conditions and Inequality 1975–1995, Report 91, Statistics Sweden, Stockholm.

McDowell, I. & Newell, C. (1987) *Measuring Health: A Guide to Rating Scales and Questionnaires*. Oxford University Press, Oxford.

Nordenfelt, L. (ed.) (1994) *Concepts and Measurement of Quality of Life in Health Care*. Kluwer, Dordrecht.

Nordenfelt, L. (1995) *On the Nature of Health: An Action-Theoretic Approach*, 2nd revised edn. Kluwer, Dordrecht.

Nordenfelt, L. (2000) *Action, Ability and Health: Essays in the Philosophy of Action and Welfare*. Kluwer, Dordrecht.

Nordenfelt, L. (2001) *Health, Science and Ordinary Language*. Rodopi Publishers, Amsterdam.

Nordenfelt, L. (2006) *Animal and Human Health and Welfare: A Philosophical Comparison*. CABI International, Wallingford.

Parsons, T. (1972) Definitions of health and illness in the light of American values and social structure. In: *Patients, Physicians, and Illness* (ed. E.G. Jaco), pp. 107–127. Free Press, New York.

Pörn, I. (1993) Health and adaptedness. *Theoretical Medicine*, **14**, 295–304.

Priorities in Health Care: Ethics, Economy, Implementation. Government Official Reports 1995:5, Stockholm.

Rendtorff, J.D. & Kemp, P. (2000) *Basic Ethical Principles in European Bioethics and Biolaw*, Vol. 1. Centre for Ethics and Law, Copenhagen.

Sandöe, P. (1999) Quality of life: three competing views. *Ethical Theory and Moral Practice*, **2**, 11–23.

Seedhouse, D. (1986) *Health: Foundations for Achievement*. John Wiley & Sons, Chichester (2nd edn 2001).

Seedhouse, D. (1988) *Ethics: The Heart of Healthcare*. John Wiley & Sons, Chichester.

Seedhouse, D. (1991) *Liberating Medicine*. John Wiley & Sons, Chichester.

Svenaeus, F. (2001) *The Hermeneutics of Medicine and the Phenomenology of Health*. Kluwer, Dordrecht.

Whitbeck, C. (1981) A theory of health. In: *Concepts of Health and Disease: Interdisciplinary Perspectives* (ed. A.L. Caplan, H.T. Engelhardt Jr & J.J. McCartney), pp. 611–626. Addison-Wesley, Reading, MA.

WHO (1948) Constitution of the World Health Organization. *Official Records of the World Health Organization*, **2**, 100.

Williams, A. (1995) *The Measurement and Valuation of Health: A Chronicle*. Centre for Health Economics, York, UK.

von Wright, G.H. (1963) *The Varieties of Goodness*. Routledge & Kegan Paul, London.

Zeiler, K. (2005) *Chosen Children: An Empirical Study and a Philosophical Analysis of Moral Aspects of Pre-Implantation Genetic Diagnosis and Germ-Line Gene Therapy*. Linköping Studies in Arts and Science, No 340, Linköping.

2. *The Concept of Dignity*

Lennart Nordenfelt

Introduction

Dignity is assumed to be a basic value (or a set of values) that a human being can possess. Moreover, it is a value that should be respected both by the person him or herself and by other human beings. Many contemporary ethicists maintain that it is of the utmost importance that such respect should be an element of health care and the care of older people.

> *I imagine my dignified old age as something that is related to respect. Dignity is the possibility of expressing opinion, the possibility of realising myself in an area which is accessible to me and the opportunity to enjoy the basic lifestyle I am used to. Not to be dependent on anybody and to have the feeling of self-realisation* (Slovak professional, Dignity and Older Europeans/Professionals, p. 17).

However, the word *dignity* is not used much in daily life. Some people even consider it to be a solemn word, a word for priests. Moreover, the concept of dignity refers to an extremely abstract property.

> *When I think about it [dignity], I find it's not an ordinary word. It might have a connection to the church and things like that. I talked to someone who said a funeral director must have dignity. He should show dignity, it's linked to that kind of situation* (34-year-old Swedish man, Dignity and Older Europeans/Young and Middle-aged People, p. 14)

> *Why do you keep coming back to dignity? It is a matter for priests* (old Slovak woman, Dignity and Older Europeans/Older People, p. 23)

Given the fact that the word dignity is not much used in ordinary speech one can wonder what role it could play in ethical codes, such as the European codes mentioned in the introduction. Is there any substantial content, or does the word have only a rhetorical function? Although I agree that there is probably an element of rhetoric, I claim that the use of the term is not empty. In the ethical documents mentioned in the preface the reference is mostly to the basic dignity common to all human beings. This is the dignity known in English as *human dignity*, often referred to by the German word

Menschenwürde. And this is the kind of dignity that has received most attention from contemporary ethicists. It is not, however, the only concept of dignity. In our ordinary speech we refer to at least three more variants of dignity. In the following I will give an introduction to all these four types: *Menschenwürde*, the dignity of merit, the dignity of moral stature and the dignity of identity. I wish to show that they all play a role in our ethical understanding of health care. (See Spiegelberg 1970 and Kolnai 1976 for excellent introductions to the modern philosophical discussion on the concept of dignity.)

2.1 The definition of dignity

2.1.1 Dictionary definitions

For the analysis of dignity it may first be useful to consult some well-respected dictionaries. In the Dignity and Older Europeans project (DOE 2004) we consulted dictionaries from six countries. All non-English definitions were translated into English by the members of the DOE project. Thus both the word to be defined (dignity) and the words that explain it were first expressed in the original language. (The presentation here is slightly simplified.)

- *The Oxford Dictionary of English*
  The English word *dignity:*
  - the quality of being worthy or honourable
  - honourable or high estate
  - an honourable office
  - a person holding an office
  - befitting elevation of aspect, manner or style
- *MSN Encarta World English Dictionary , North American Edition*
  The English word *dignity:*
  - pride and self-respect
  - seriousness in behaviour
  - worthiness
  - due respect
  - high office
  - dignitary
- *Nouveau Petit Robert, dictionnaire alphabétique et analogique de la langue française*
  The French word *dignité:*
  - function, title or charge that gives to someone an eminent rank
  - respect that someone merits
  - self-respect
  - appearance and behaviour that translate this feeling
- *Nationalencyklopedins ordbok*
  The Swedish word *värdighet:*
  - sense of what is worthy behaviour
  - being worthy
  - high position and honour

- *Słownik Języka Polskiego*
  . The Polish noun *godność:*
  - being aware of one's own value, self-respect; honour, pride; to have a feeling of dignity
  - honourable position, office, title, function
  - family name
  the Polish adjective *godny:*
  - worthy of something
  - someone who is full of a feeling of his or her own worth
  - dignified conduct or behaviour
- *Velký sociologický slovník*
  The Czech word *dustojnos:*
  - Attribute of high social prestige. Dignity is associated with respect and reverence on the part of the surrounding community. The acknowledged sign of dignity is serious, consistent and gentle behaviour, showing signs of wisdom and justice. Dignity is traditionally attributed to old age and important social status.
  - Awareness of own dignity that may or may not be perceived by those around. This awareness plays an important role in inner integration of personality. Preservation of dignity is enabled by the person's effective defence against social humiliation and derision. The right to this personal dignity belongs to civil and human rights. The personal dignity is relative. Various societies have their own model of dignity associated with values of the social group or society.
- *Krátky slovník slovenského jazyka*
  The Slovak adjective *dostojnost:*
  - revered
  - serious, noble
  - appropriate, suitable
- *Diccionario de la Lengua Española*
  The Spanish word *dignidad:*
  - quality of a dignified person
  - excellence, enhancement
  - seriousness and propriety in behaviour
  - honourable post or job
  - any of the qualities which characterise a prestigious post, such as a deanery
  - person who embodies one of these qualities
  - archbishop or bishop
  - the post of Grand Master

2.1.2 Comments on the dictionary definitions

I will here summarise some of the most common connotations of dignity according to the dictionaries.

High office, honourable post or occupation

This is probably the oldest use of the word *dignity* mentioned in classical texts (the Latin *dignitas*).

Person holding a high office

In English the word *dignitary* also exists (in Swedish the old word *dignitär* has the same sense), which perhaps more precisely denotes a person holding a high office, especially in church or government. The term *dignidad* in Spanish can have very special connotations in this direction, such as archbishop, bishop or Grand Master of a religious order.

The quality of being worthy

There are various similar expressions for this notion. 'Worthiness' or 'the state or quality of being worthy of honour' as well as 'excellence' are common synonyms.

Respect

Respect is an important notion but also a difficult one. It is clear that in some languages respect is a synonym for dignity. Taken literally, this would mean that dignity is interpreted as an attitude. But who, then, is the possessor of dignity? Is it the subject (the person who respects) or the object (the person respected)? The Czech explanation indicates that it must be the object. 'Dignity is associated with respect and reverence on the part of the surrounding community.' 'Respect that someone deserves' is also mentioned in some dictionaries.

Self-respect

A similar question arises here: self-respect is mentioned as a synonym of dignity in several of the dictionaries.

In the Polish dictionary self-respect is explained as awareness of one's own value. This is quite similar to the Czech 'awareness of own dignity which may not be perceived by those around'. The English 'sense of self-importance' meaning being full of oneself is similar but has distinctly negative connotations.

In this case there seems to be an identification of dignity with an attitude or a cognition. A person has dignity if the person respects him or herself. But here, in contradistinction to the case of respect pure and simple, there is no trouble in identifying the possessor of dignity. The subject and object are identical.

Seriousness of behaviour

This is an idea common to many of the languages. The expressions can vary a little: 'befitting elevation of aspect, manner or style' (*Oxford English Dictionary*) 'a formal, stately or grave bearing' (*Collins English Dictionary*) and 'seriousness and propriety in behaviour' (the Spanish dictionary). In the French dictionary this behaviour is assumed to reflect the subject's self-respect. It says: 'appearance and behaviour that translates the feeling [of self-respect]'.

It appears, therefore, that there is a great overlap in the senses of the European words that are traditionally translated into the English 'dignity'. Nevertheless there are some interesting differences in emphasis, and some idiosyncratic uses, such as the Polish use of the term in the sense of 'family name'. On the whole, however, we can find some common ground which includes the concepts of high office, the quality of being worthy, respect and self-respect.

In proceeding to a further analysis and explication of the concept of dignity I will have these different dictionary definitions in mind. Most of the senses of dignity mentioned in the list above will influence this analysis. An exception is the sense where the word denotes a person holding an office. The underlying abstract connotation, dignity as a high office or rank, however, is the prototype for what we call the *dignity of merit*. In the general analysis I have not limited myself to any specific office or rank. The idea has been generalised to all kinds of ranks, formal as well as informal. I have particularly stressed the *value* of a position rather than the position itself.

2.2   Dignity: towards an analysis

2.2.1   Introduction

In the following analysis I will distinguish four concepts of dignity and spell out their differences. This analysis is inspired partly by the linguistic analysis just presented, but partly also by observations in the scholarly literature on dignity. The four concepts are: the dignity of merit, the dignity of moral or existential stature, the dignity of identity and the universal human dignity (*Menschenwürde*). The dignity of merit depends on social rank and position. There are many types of this kind of dignity, and it is very unevenly distributed among human beings. The dignity of moral stature is the result of the moral deeds of the subject; it can be reduced or lost through immoral actions. This kind of dignity is tied to the idea of a dignified character and of dignity as a virtue. The dignity of identity is tied to the integrity of the subject's body and mind, and in many instances, although not always, it is also dependent on the subject's self-image. *Menschenwürde* pertains to all human beings to the same extent, and cannot be lost as long as a person exists.

2.2.2   The common core

The four types of dignity have some important properties in common. Consider the following:

- 'Dignity' refers to a special dimension of value. In the case of *Menschenwürde* there is only one position on that scale, but with the other kinds of dignity people can have different positions on the scale; they can be either more or less dignified.
- The dignity of a person is worthy of respect from others and from the person him or herself.
- The dignity has a ground, normally a set of properties, belonging to the subject.

In many cases the dignity of a person confers a set of rights on that person. Paying respect to the dignity then means respecting the rights of the subject. In some cases paying respect can also be expressed simply by thinking highly of the person or of the qualities of the person.

2.2.3   The four concepts of dignity
Dignity as merit

> *I think you deserve dignity if you have done something good or in a way worked your way up for it* (18-year-old Swedish woman, Dignity and Older Europeans/Young and Middle-aged People, p.15).

30

A person who has a rank or holds an office that entails a set of rights has a special dignity. This is probably the oldest sense of the Latin *dignitas*, which was used with reference to excellence and distinction, properties typically pertaining to senators and other people of high rank in Roman society. This sense of the word is still current in the romance languages: the Spanish word *dignidad* can refer to a person of a high rank, in particular in the clerical hierarchy, such as an archbishop.

We may refer to this dignity as dignity of merit, although in some cases a person may be born with such a dignity, as in the case of a hereditary monarchy. Thus, for example, a king, a cabinet minister, a bishop and a doctor have special dignities of merit that come with their positions. These are the *formal dignities of merit*. Typically, as the term implies, these dignities of merit are bestowed upon people through some formal act, for instance an appointment.

The dignity of merit is also related to the notions of rights and respect. The cabinet minister, the bishop and the doctor have rights attached to their positions. These rights should be respected by those who approach the people in question.

We may also acknowledge some *informal dignities of merit*, where people have earned general merit through their deeds and deserve respect for this. The achievements of artists, scientists and athletes are often acknowledged and highly regarded. Normally, the people in question cannot claim any formal rights but they are often treated as if they had such rights.

It is significant that the dignities of merit can come and go. People can be promoted, but they can also be demoted. People can have an informal fame and a great reputation for some time, but they can lose it quite suddenly. Another feature of the dignities of merit is that they admit of degrees. Most positions, professional or otherwise, are ordered in hierarchies. A general is higher on the military scale than a sergeant; a bishop is higher on the clerical scale than a parish priest.

A special dignity of merit may be attributed to older people. This is the wisdom of older people, comprising what they have been able to extract from all their experiences in life.

The concept [of dignity] is often connected to people with experience and people with a special dignity … those who have accomplished something in society (57-year-old Swedish man, Dignity and Older Europeans/Young and Middle-aged People, p. 20).

Dignity as moral stature: a dignity tied to self-respect

Dignified behaviour is when you don't try to be superior to others … not patronising other people (18-year-old Swedish woman, Dignity and Older Europeans/Young and Middle-aged People, p. 18).

You can say that you get dignity by treating others with respect (an 18-year-old Swedish woman, Dignity and Older Europeans/Young and Middle-aged People, p. 16).

Dignity is to respect the convictions of the person. The religious convictions, they are part of our life and it's important (French nurse, Dignity and Older Europeans/Professionals, p. 25).

31

I shall now turn to the dignity of moral stature, a type of dignity that has some features in common with the general dignity of merit. It is, one might say, a dignity of quite a special kind of merit. This is a dignity that is very much dependent upon the thoughts and deeds of the subject. We sometimes talk about a dignified character as a personality disposed to respect the moral law. Related to this is the idea that *dignified conduct* is action in accordance with the moral law.

Sometimes the idea of dignified conduct is tied to actions of exceptional moral value, for instance in the face of extreme adversity or where the price paid is high. In extreme circumstances the price can be one's own life. Some famous people in history have actually sacrificed their lives in order to preserve their dignity. One of these was the philosopher Socrates, who was sentenced to death for the alleged crime of having seduced the youth of Athens. In prison Socrates drank a cup of poison and died in the company of some of his pupils. He thought that he would not have retained his dignity if he had escaped from his imprisonment, which would in fact have been quite possible for him to do.

Like most ordinary dignities of merit, the dignity of moral stature is dimensional in that it can vary from an extremely high level to an extremely low one. The degree of dignity can be high or low depending upon the moral value of one's actions. There is an important difference, however, between the dignities of merit and the dignity of moral stature in that the latter does not provide the subject with any rights. A prime minister or a general has certain rights attached to the position they hold. But a highly moral person does not acquire any rights through his or her actions. In fact, it is an interesting feature of morality that the moral value of an action would be lost or at least diminished if it were to result in certain rights or privileges for the subject.

This observation has consequences for the notion of respect as tied to moral stature. Respect is related to morality in several ways. First, the moral agent pays respect to others. This is a central feature of morality itself. Part of the sense of being moral is to respect other people's rights, either the special rights bestowed upon them by legal authorities or the specifically human rights that all people have (to be discussed below). But, second, there is a special respect that the moral agents deserve, but one that is not tied to any of their rights. We ought to pay respect to moral agents in the sense of thinking highly and speaking well of them.

A third way in which respect enters the dignity of moral stature is as *self-respect*.

In order to be able to show other people respect I think you have to learn to respect yourself first (19-year-old Swedish man, Dignity and Older Europeans/Young and Middle-aged People, p. 21).

We usually talk about this in a negative mode, e.g. we say that we cannot respect ourselves if we betray our country or let our people down. Socrates could not keep his self-respect if he did not choose the moral route. I think this indicates that self-respect is a threshold notion. If one remains a moral agent, then one can keep one's self-respect. One will not end up despising oneself. It is not, however, a feature of moral agents to think very highly of themselves as a result of particular moral 'achievements'. This would turn the self-respect into pride or self-satisfaction, attitudes which are alien to the moral stance. (See the analysis made by Szawarski 1986.)

32

I have suggested that self-respect is a threshold concept, but it does not follow from this that it is not dimensional. On the negative side one can respect oneself less and less, depending on the varying degrees of negative value that one's actions have. To have dignity, then, could mean possessing a certain moral standard. This kind of dignity can have degrees: one's moral standard can be high or low, or it may not even reach the minimal threshold.

The dignity of identity
I will now turn to a kind of dignity that is not dependent on the subject's merits, be they formal or informal or having to do with moral status. This kind of dignity is quite difficult to define, although it is probably the most important sense in the contexts of illness or ageing. It is significant of this kind of dignity that it can be taken from us by external events, by the acts of other people as well as by injury, illness and old age.

> *They [older people] are de-individualised, that's not dignity, they are treated like children in a day nursery* (52-year-old Swedish man, Dignity and Older Europeans/Young and Middle-aged People, p. 23).

> *If someone is sat on the commode and they are completely naked, you don't leave the door wide open. You might have a woman on the commode and you have got a man next door and you don't know when they are going to come out of their rooms. I certainly wouldn't want to be seen by my neighbour* (British care assistant, Dignity and Older Europeans/Professionals, p. 32).

> *The permanent staff who are working there all the time, and probably are really bored with their job, they show the least dignified behaviour towards older people. We part-timers wonder how they can say such things. I have found that the ordinary staff treat older people as objects* (26-year-old Swedish nursing assistant, Dignity and Older Europeans/Young and Middle-aged People, p. 23).

I will tentatively call this the *dignity of identity*. It is the dignity that we attach to ourselves as integrated and autonomous persons, with a history and a future, with all our relationships to other human beings. Most of us have a basic respect for our own identity, although it need not be in any way remarkable from a moral or other point of view. But this self-respect can easily be shattered, for instance by nature itself, in illness and the disability of illness and old age, but also by the cruelty of other people.

Humiliation can be even more profound when it is the result of intentional cruelty. Statman (2000, p. 528) has reflected on this phenomenon in an insightful way:

> That other people can hit me, put me in jail and ridicule me publicly is beyond question. But why should such behaviors be taken as constituting a reason for me to respect myself less? How could it ever be rational to consider my *self*-respect injured because of the disrespect other people express toward me?

And he goes on to say (p. 534):

> Though the victim of humiliation often does not value the standards of worthiness and of social success assumed by the humiliator, the humiliator manages to shatter

the victim's self-respect, to make her feel unworthy, diminished in stature, devalued.

There is some kind of paradox here. How can humiliation rob me of my dignity? How can I lose my dignity when I am attacked by people whose moral views I despise? The humiliation is not (normally) a case of formal demotion. The perpetrators cannot (normally) do anything about my formal or informal merits. Nor can they by their immoral acts rob me of my moral stature. This can only happen if they succeed in provoking me to react in an immoral way. So if there is a case of dignity here, it is neither the dignity of merit nor the dignity of moral stature. It must be a dignity attached to the person's integrity and identity as a human being. (See Kolnai 1976 for similar observations.)

The interesting psychological truth here is that people's feeling of worth is to a great extent tied to how they are looked upon by other people, irrespective of the nature of the values held by these people. The inhuman treatment entails some kind of social exclusion – the SS officer by his brutal acts tells the prisoner: you do not belong to us, we are the elite – and this social exclusion is humiliating even if one does not in the least adhere to the values of (in the given example) the SS officer. This psychological fact has to be accepted, despite the long tradition of the Stoics and the long religious traditions that have taught us to ignore unjust acts directed against us.

But is dignity in this sense, then, identical with a *feeling* or *sense* of worth? If we are only talking about a psychological fact, i.e. the self-confidence or self-respect of the person, then there is perhaps no need for a special concept of dignity.

I will here argue the case for an objective (or at least inter-subjective) dignity of identity. Cruel people can succeed in certain things apart from humiliating us. They can intrude into our private sphere, can physically hurt us, and can restrict our autonomy in many ways, for instance by putting us in jail. All these changes are extra-psychological. They do not just entail feelings of worthlessness or of humiliation. Intrusion in the private sphere is a violation of the person's integrity. Hurting a person is not only violation of integrity; it also entails a change in the person's identity. After this experience, the victim becomes a person with a trauma: in a salient sense, this is a new physical identity. Autonomy can be tampered with, when people are prevented from doing what they want to do or are entitled to do. Finally, insulting, hurting or hindering people entails excluding them from one's community.

Thus the factors that form the basis of the dignity of identity are the subjects' integrity and autonomy, including their social relations. These factors are typically associated with a sense of integrity and autonomy. And when a person's integrity and autonomy are tampered with, this is typically associated with a *feeling* of humiliation or loss of self-respect on the part of the subject. Self-respect is thus an important concept in connection also with the dignity of identity.

One example, crystal-clear, of unworthy behaviour is when you are unworthy towards yourself. I don't know how to express it right but if you are really self-destructive, for instance, maybe that's the best example (17-year-old Swedish man, Dignity and Older Europeans/ Young and Middle-aged People, p. 24).

Thus, as in the case of dignity of moral stature, self-respect is often tied to the dignity of identity. One can respect the fact that one's identity is undamaged or even improved, and one can lose one's self-respect when one's identity has been broken down. Again, as in the case of moral stature, this self-respect does not entail the respect of any special rights pertaining to the individual. There are, for instance, no rights that have been violated by nature when older people gradually lose their autonomy or when a car accident deforms an individual's body.

It is another matter, which may be a source of confusion, that we all also have some basic rights (in relation to our fellow human beings) with regard to integrity and autonomy. These rights are grounded in another dignity, the dignity of *Menschenwürde*, to be discussed below.

2.2.4 Axel Honneth's theory of respect

In general, self-awareness and feelings are strongly connected to the dignity of identity. An author who has studied this phenomenon with particular care is the German philosopher Axel Honneth (1992). Honneth has created a theory of dignity (although it explicitly deals with the notion of respect) where feelings play a fundamental part. The most crucial concept is perhaps self-perception or, more generally, *having an image of oneself* as a person. Here I must limit myself to summarising Honneth's distinctions, first between three forms of disrespect, then, in parallel, between three positive variants of respect and thereby dignity. Consider first the three forms of disrespect.

Honneth says that it is obvious that we use the terms *disrespect* and *insult* in everyday language to designate a variety of degrees of psychological injury to a subject. The differences between these forms are measured 'by the degree to which they can upset a person's practical relationship to self by depriving this person of the recognition of certain claims to identity' (p. 190). The first type of disrespect pertains to a person's physical integrity. Any form of practical maltreatment that forcibly deprives someone of any opportunity to dispose freely of their own body represents the most fundamental type of personal degradation and does lasting damage to the subject's confidence.

Disrespect that interrupts the continuity of a positive image of a person's self even at the corporeal level is to be distinguished from forms of degradation that affect a person's normative understanding of him or herself.

> Should the person be systematically denied certain rights (to participate in the institutional order), the implication is that he or she is not deemed to possess the same degree of moral accountability as other members of society. ... For the individual, having socially valid rights withheld from him or her signifies a violation of the person's intersubjective expectation that he or she will be recognized as a subject capable of reaching moral judgments (p. 191).

This second type of disrespect must be set off from a third type of degradation, which entails negative consequences for the social value of individuals or groups.

> Only when we consider these evaluative forms of disrespect, namely, the denigration of individual or collective life-styles, do we actually arrive at the form of behaviour for which our everyday language provides such designations as 'insult' or

'degradation'. The honour, dignity or status of a person can be understood to signify the degree of social acceptance forthcoming for a person's method of self-realization within the horizon of cultural traditions within a society (p. 191).

Individuals who experience this type of social devaluation typically lose their self-esteem – they are no longer in a position to conceive of themselves as beings whose characteristic traits and abilities are worthy of esteem.

The differentiation of the three forms of disrespect provides us with a key to classifying the positive counterparts, i.e. as Honneth says, relationships of mutual recognition.

1 Body-related self-confidence; body-related sense of security in expressing one's own needs and feelings. The key concepts here are love and *self-confidence*.
2 The positive attitude that subjects can assume towards themselves if they experience legal recognition is that of fundamental self-respect. The key concepts are rights and *self-respect*.
3 Relationship of recognition that can aid the individual in acquiring self-esteem. The key concepts are solidarity and *self-esteem*.

This analysis shows that feelings such as self-confidence, self-respect and self-esteem play a central part in forming our identity. When our identity is infringed or even threatened, we typically feel degraded or humiliated and lose our self-confidence, self-respect or self-esteem. I also believe that our *idea* of personal identity is dependent on the notion of feeling and, more specifically, the notion of self-image.

2.2.5 More on dignity of identity
Having paid this necessary tribute to the notion of feeling, I think nevertheless that we must admit that dignity need not always be tied to the subject's self-image. This is particularly not so with *Menschenwürde*, which by hypothesis is there as long as a human being exists, conscious or unconscious. But a dignity of merit may also be there without the subject acknowledging it. A person may just have been promoted to a position without knowing about it, for instance. And certainly a person may be dignified in a moral sense without being aware of it, or without particularly thinking about it. Below I will argue that even the dignity of identity may exist without the subject's awareness of it. Of course, in most cases people are *typically* aware of their dignity, but there is no necessary connection.

So far I have only considered the case where a person's self-respect has diminished or been lost as a result of another person's disrespectful acts. But the identity version of dignity is relevant also in cases when we say that illness, impairment, disability and old age can rob one of one's dignity. What could happen in such cases?

To some extent we already know the answers. When one's face has been badly damaged in a car accident, one's physical identity has been shattered. When one has lost one's legs, one's physical identity is radically transformed and one's autonomy is greatly diminished. A disabled person is almost by definition a person with restricted autonomy, and restricted autonomy normally entails exclusion from some communities.

Older people are often subject to illness and disability. For older people there is the additional burden that their disability is often irreversible. They believe or know that they will remain disabled for the rest of their life. Their identity is permanently and drastically changed.

Well, they have lost a lot of self-esteem and dignity just through having the stroke anyway, so if we can make them feel what they are capable of doing then you can progress on that and help them (British professional, Dignity and Older Europeans/Professionals, p. 29).

In the context of the Home project, Franklin et al. (2006) studied this phenomenon particularly with regard to old age in an interview study of nursing home residents. A powerful experience among these older people was that they were no longer able to control their bodily functions. This recognition was a threat to their self-image and identity. 'Losing different bodily functions meant an almost inevitable dependency that the elderly people experienced as violating and difficult to handle despite their reconciliation with their situation on another level' (p. 138).

It's horrible not being able to take care of myself. I can always get help but it's horrible to wake up when you wet on your own bed. Everything you do you're dependent on others. For example, when you need to go to the toilet. It doesn't feel good to ask for help going to the toilet, just like babies (Franklin et al. 2006, p. 138).

A common consequence of such disabilities relating to old age is that the people around them change their attitudes towards older people:

You see … it feels as if they treat us as if we don't understand anything even though we have lived a whole life (Franklin et al. 2006, p. 139).

When I lost my hearing people started to ignore me. They didn't treat me as a human being any more and when I lost my eyesight there was nothing left (Franklin et al. 2006, p. 139).

There is also a noticeable change in the appearance of older people (and some ill people). For some individuals this marks an extremely painful change of identity. A beautiful woman, whose identity has literally consisted of her beauty, is gradually transformed through ageing into a much less attractive person. Likewise, an athlete, whose fame is wholly dependent on achievements on the track, is gradually transformed into a weak, disabled person who is excluded from his previous community.

Disability and restricted autonomy have a further consequence for a person's identity and thereby dignity. The care of ill people and older people who cannot move about and take care of themselves is relegated to other people, the carers. The risk of intrusion into one's private sphere, i.e. of a violation of one's integrity, then becomes high.

A particular kind of handicap is a consequence of the development of society. Rapid technological progress, in particular the prevalence of information technology, leaves older people behind. They have not been trained to use such technologies and as a result they encounter difficulties in doing routine things such as paying bills.

That must be an aspect of a really undignified life. Suddenly you can't manage in society any more, not because you have become frail, but because society has run away from you, so to speak. So you can't pay your bills any more without using the Internet (27-year-old Swedish woman, Dignity and Older Europeans/Young and Middle-aged People, p. 34)

Consider further the case of individuals who are unconscious or in the late stages of senile dementia. They are not aware of what is happening around them. Nevertheless, we would say that their dignity could be violated. They could be treated disrespectfully, and unfortunately they often are. This disrespect is not noticed by the client, who does not suffer for this reason. The assumption of an objective identity allows us to explain why the dignity of the client is still violated. For example, the carer may have left the client naked for some time so that they could be seen by others. Then the client's privacy and integrity have been tampered with.

We may pursue this line of thought even to the dead (see Chapter 8). It is possible, I think, to violate the dignity of dead people, by slandering them or by spitting on their grave. In this case the violation cannot be understood unless there is an objective ground for the dignity.

And dignity does not just concern living human beings but also when you're dead (Swedish professional, Dignity and Older Europeans/ Professionals, p. 16).

I feel that when somebody has passed away their dignity is in some way enhanced; therefore I get even more humble and feel even more respect for them (Swedish professional, Dignity and Older Europeans/ Professionals, p. 16).

Indeed, in an obvious sense the dead person does not exist as a person. There is, however, still something to be revered and respected. There is a dead body and there is a memory of the live person that we wish to respect.

2.2.6 Human dignity (*Menschenwürde*)

But every human being has a fundamental dignity just by being a human being. So we talk about Menschenwürde *and in that case, irrespective of how we act, it is a fundamental value, which is invaluable as such; you have it because you are a human being* (25-year-old Swedish woman, Dignity and older Europeans/Young and Middle-aged People, p. 47).

It defines humanity, it's a universal value (French nurse, Dignity and older Europeans/ Professionals, p. 24).

So far I have introduced three notions of dignity, which are quite different but have two important features in common. First, people can have these types of dignity to various extents. Some people have high degrees of dignity, have a high rank in some hierarchy, have a high moral standard and have an undamaged identity. Others score low along these dimensions, and we can also have combinations where a person has a high degree of dignity along one scale and a low one along another. Second, all these three types of dignity can come and go. A person can move from one point on a scale to another, be promoted at one time and demoted at another. One's moral status can rise and decline, and one's identity can be shattered and restored. With regard to the dignity of merit in particular, one can even be completely removed from a scale and have no merit whatsoever.

One kind of dignity is completely different in these important respects. *Human dignity*, sometimes referred to by the German term *Menschenwürde*, refers to a kind of dignity that we all have as humans, or are assumed to have just because we are humans. This is the specifically human value. We all have this value to the same degree, i.e. we are equal with respect to this kind of dignity; *Menschenwürde* cannot be taken from human beings as long as they are alive.

Given our equal human dignity, no one may be treated with less respect than anyone else with regard to basic human rights. The respect entails at least a fulfilment of the rights that are attached to the dignity in question. It is the duty of all of us to respect all these rights. In particular, an older person has the same basic human rights as a young person.

The idea of an equal human value is now common and accepted in the civilised world. It is a cornerstone of most religions and it has an important place in Western secular ideology. The United Nations has attempted to capture this notion in its *Declaration of Human Rights*. The first article of the *Universal Declaration of Human Rights* (1948) states: 'All human beings are born free, equal in dignity and human rights. They are endowed with reason and conscience and should act towards one another in a spirit of brotherhood.'

In philosophical discussions about human rights it is common to regard a few of these rights as basic and the others as derived. Birnbacher (1996) gives the following four as the minimal human rights: (1) provision of the necessary means of existence, (2) freedom from severe and continual pain, (3) minimal liberty and (4) minimal self-respect. The UN Declaration, however, provides a more comprehensive list and includes, for instance, the right to a nationality, the right to own property and the right to education.

But what is the ground for *Menschenwürde*? What is it about humans as a species that gives them a high dignity? One answer is the traditional Christian one: humans were created in God's image. The common modern answer, inspired by Kant, refers instead to capacities crucial to humans. The first is consciousness and the ability to think, i.e. our reason. This includes the power of self-consciousness. Human beings can reflect upon themselves. Second, human beings are different from other creatures in the world through not being determinate. They are free to decide their own way of life. Pico della Mirandola in the 16th century described how God the Father gave humans an indeterminate nature (1948, p. 227).

But if there is no predetermined goal in Nature, then the human being must also be the creator of norms and values. This is the third element in human dignity, i.e. autonomy, most clearly explicated by Kant: 'Autonomy is thus the basis of the dignity of both human nature and of every rational nature' (*Groundwork of the Metaphysics of Morals* (1997), p. 53).

In short, *Menschenwürde* is a dignity belonging to every human being to the same degree throughout life. It cannot be taken away from anyone and it cannot be attributed to any creature by fiat. This human dignity is the ground for specifically human rights. (For a further discussion of human dignity and its grounds, see sections 2.3 and 2.5 below.)

2.2.7 Concluding remarks

To summarise this presentation of four kinds of dignity:

- *Human dignity* pertains to all human beings to the same extent and cannot be lost as long as the individuals exist.
- The *dignity of merit* depends on social rank and formal positions in life. There are many types of this kind of dignity and it is very unevenly distributed among human beings. The dignity of merit exists in degrees and it can come and go.
- The *dignity of moral stature* is the result of the moral deeds of the subject; it can be reduced or lost through immoral deeds. This kind of dignity is tied to the idea of a dignified character and of dignity as a virtue. The dignity of moral stature is a dignity of degree and it is also unevenly distributed among humans.
- The *dignity of identity* is tied to the integrity of the subject's body and mind, and in many instances, although not always, it is also dependent on the subject's self-image. This dignity can come and go as a result of the deeds of fellow human beings and also as a result of changes in the subject's body and mind.

2.3 *Relationships between the notions of dignity*

2.3.1 On the relation between dignity of identity and human dignity

It is interesting to inquire into the relationships between the various types of dignity that have been sketched here. Consider the relationship between the dignity of identity and human dignity. How distinct are they and how important is it to distinguish between them? On the face of it they partly deal with the same matters. The reasons for protecting the dignity of identity seem to lie close to the reasons for protecting human dignity. Moreover, both kinds of dignity are grounded on basic human properties such as the conditions for life and autonomy.

It is also clear from my analysis that violating human dignity is often tantamount to violating the dignity of identity. When *A* is cruel to *B* and does not respect *B*'s integrity then *A* violates both *B*'s human dignity and his or her dignity of identity. Conversely, to respect human dignity is at the same time to respect a person's dignity of identity. What, then, is the reason for distinguishing between the two?

There are at least four features that distinguish human dignity from dignity of identity and which I wish to underline here. The first two, and perhaps most crucial, are the ones mentioned in my summary above. Human dignity is fixed once and for all and it is the same for all people. The dignity of identity can vary between people and it can vary over time. The person who says, 'I lost my dignity when my face was deformed in the car accident', must be talking of dignity of identity. Human dignity can, by hypothesis, not be lost.

A third distinguishing feature is embedded in my example above. Human dignity, like dignity of identity, can be violated by individuals and collectives of human beings, such as political parties and states. But unlike dignity of identity, human dignity cannot be violated by nature itself. Car accidents and natural phenomena, on the other hand, may rob individuals of their dignity of identity. I highlighted earlier how diseases and the degenerative processes of old age can result in a deformation of a person's body and mind, with a reduction or even loss of dignity as a further result. Fourthly, our common discourse suggests that even the dead can have a dignity that can be violated and tampered with (see Chapter 8). Human dignity (*Menschenwürde*), on the other hand, is tied to the living human being.

2.3.2 Dependencies among the varieties of dignity

The various kinds of dignity are dependent on each other. The dignity of moral stature is particularly tied to the subject's activities. An important interpretation of 'acting in a dignified way' is acting morally in a certain way. A crucial part of such dignified moral activity is to pay respect to other people by thinking highly of them, by recognising their identity or by fulfilling their rights. Thus a morally dignified person, the person who acts in a dignified way, pays respect to other people's human dignity, their dignity of identity or at times their dignity of merit. For an illustration of such dependency, see the analysis of the French DOE report in Chapter 9.

It can be noted that the dignity of moral stature is particularly highlighted when the bearer is in a *subject* (or agentive) position. The other dignities are particularly high-lighted as *objects of respect.*

2.3.3 Relations between dignity and some other human values

In this section I will connect my analysis of dignity to the other central human values discussed at the beginning of this chapter.

Dignity, autonomy and integrity

There is a particularly close relationship between dignity, on the one hand, and auton-omy and integrity on the other. In the discussion about the dignity of identity I noted that a person's autonomy and integrity are fundamental elements of their identity. To respect the person's autonomy and integrity is to respect crucial parts of their identity. Likewise, in most conceptions of human dignity individuals' right to decide for them-selves (i.e. their right to autonomy), and their right to have their bodies and properties intact, are included as basic rights.

Thus autonomy and integrity are parts of the identity of a person. This identity in turn has, as I have claimed, a special value, a dignity. Hence the autonomy and integrity of the person partly constitute the dignity of identity of the person.

People's basic rights, determined by their human dignity, also pertain to autonomy and integrity. A difference between human dignity and identity lies in the fact that human dignity determines a basic platform that is universal for all people. What is required in terms of autonomy and integrity in the case of identity, in order for full dignity to be preserved, will differ from person to person. The difference is partly dependent on the individual's own interpretation of the situation, their self-confidence, self-respect and self-esteem.

The distinction between dignity and quality of life

What is the relation between dignity and quality of life? Is quality of life a part of dignity, is it a cause or is it an effect? In several of the empirical reports from the DOE project one could find statements of the following kind: 'Satisfaction with life appeared to be key in relation to experiencing dignity in the lives of these older people.' And also: 'Inner contentment appeared to participants to be an expression of dignity' (Slovakia, Older People, pp. 10–12). The question to be asked here is: Do these people genuinely consider dignity (in one of its senses) to be identical with subjective quality of life or satisfaction with life? Or is there a risk that we, as interpreters, wrongly come to this conclusion?

Luckily there is a further interpretation that is probably the most reasonable in many instances. Satisfaction with life may be a sign that dignity is there, without satisfaction with life being identical with (or constituting) dignity. Moreover, the results seem to show that satisfaction concerns one's personal life in general; people do not refer to any old pleasure or just a good laugh and call that dignity. Dignity, or the feeling of dignity, seems to be related to an enduring state of affairs attached to one's person. This feeling leads to or involves also satisfaction with life. Such an interpretation is plausible and does not contradict anything in our theoretical model.

Quality of life may be both a cause and an effect of dignity or a sense of dignity. Individuals who are happy can as a result of their happiness have self-confidence, self-respect and self-esteem. Thus the level of their dignity of identity can be raised and maintained. But the converse relation is perhaps the most plausible. People who feel confident and who respect themselves both as moral beings and as whole integrated beings will, other things being equal, be happy. Therefore happiness can often be an expression of dignity.

2.4 Further explorations on dignity. A commentary on some other authors

2.4.1 On intrinsic and attributed dignity: Daniel Sulmasy

Before leaving this exploration of dignity I wish to call attention to two interesting articles by the American philosopher Daniel Sulmasy (1997, 2006). In these articles Sulmasy introduces the distinction between dignity as an intrinsic property and dignity as an attributed property. In Sulmasy (2006) he introduces some further concepts pertaining to dignity, namely the concepts of instrumental, attributed and derivative values. Here I will focus on the first distinction, the one between intrinsic and attributed values.

Sulmasy's basic idea is that what I here call human dignity is an intrinsic value. His definition runs: 'Dignity is a value that everyone has simply because he or she is human, it is something that everyone has equally, and that it is inalienable' (1997, p. 19). He calls it the Kantian/Catholic perspective. The intrinsic aspect of human dignity is, he says, given in every human encounter. In the later article Sulmasy argues forcefully for the idea that the intrinsic dignity is dependent on the notion of natural kinds. Intrinsic value, he says, is the value that something has solely in virtue of its being the kind of thing it is (2006, p. 74).

On the other hand, Sulmasy says:

the second broad type of dignity is attributed dignity. This is not a value or worth that one has by virtue of being human, but a value or worth that one acquires by virtue of some attribution of worth, either by oneself or others. Examples include the dignity of rank, the dignity of self-esteem, the dignity of reserve, of seriousness, of one's standing in the community, the dignity of honour or esteem from others, and the dignity that one attributes to oneself or others by virtue of certain capacities or accomplishments (1997, p. 19).

It appears that Sulmasy calls every form of dignity other than human dignity an attributed dignity. He includes here what I have called dignity of merit (consider his dignity of rank, of one's standing in the community, of honour or esteem) and at least elements of what I call dignity of identity (self-esteem and the dignity that one attributes to oneself by virtue of certain capacities or accomplishments). In a later passage on dignity and control it becomes evident that Sulmasy would include some of the further features that I have mentioned with regard to dignity of identity. 'For many, dignity is equated with being in control. Losing one's valued independence, through the limitations imposed by disease … seems to mean the loss of dignity. I do not deny that loss of control means loss of attributed dignity' (1997, p. 21). Sulmasy does not particularly recognise what I have called dignity of moral stature, although it may be included in his dignity of self-esteem.

Sulmasy does not pursue the analysis of the notion of attributed dignity beyond making the contrast with human dignity. His terminological choice is a challenge, however, for further analysis in order to deepen our understanding of the nature of dignities. What could we mean by an attributed dignity? Are all dignities apart from human dignity really attributed in the lexical sense of the word? And could not human dignity be regarded as attributed?

It is easy to see that attribution makes sense in the paradigm cases of dignity of merit, the dignity accompanying a high position or rank. I noted above that a specific act of appointment is often presupposed when a person acquires a high position or rank. The government appoints high officials; the archbishop appoints other bishops and priests, etc. However, even within the category of dignity of merit we encounter difficulties. Some positions are hereditary: a king can be born a king, with no need for somebody to appoint him. This specific case is perhaps not so troublesome and may be countered in the following way. Even if the king can be born a king, his dynasty has at some stage been selected by some of his fellow-countrymen. At a certain time in history some attribution must have been made.

But what about unofficial merit? Indeed, there may be an unofficial attribution. Honour or esteem is something that by definition issues from other people. However, honour does not presuppose any specific *act* of attribution. On the other hand, honour and esteem presuppose an *attitude* on the part of the people around the subject.

But what about dignity as moral stature and the dignity of identity? There is first a distinction to be made between dignity as acquired through an achievement (moral or otherwise) and dignity as attributed through some kind of act, decision or, for that matter, attitude. I would say that a person may have the dignity of moral stature without anyone, even the subject, believing or acknowledging this. It would be misleading to say that the subject through his or her moral deeds has attributed to him or herself the dignity of moral stature; rather, the subject has achieved or acquired the dignity.

But could one not say that there must be some recognition of the subject's dignity of moral stature for it to exist? And is not this recognition a kind of attribution of the dignity? No, it would be absurd to say that the morality of a person is dependent on other people's acknowledgement. The ground for the dignity, I contend, is the moral status itself, not the recognition of it by other people. It would in general be impossible to uphold the idea that recognition is necessary for dignity (apart from the cases of honour and esteem where this is true by definition). In the basic case of human dignity it is crucial that human dignity exists even if nobody around the subject would acknowledge the fact.

So, in the case of moral dignity, even if some action is presupposed for the existence of dignity, this is not an act of attribution but rather an act of achievement. We may therefore distinguish between *acquired* dignity and attributed dignity.

Consider now the dignity of identity. Is this a dignity that is attributed by someone? It is initially plausible to contend that the subject attributes this dignity to him or herself. The subject has a picture of the self and typically recognises when this picture is shattered. Is the dignity of identity not then attributed by the subject?

My answer to this difficult question is that the subject has contributed substantially to the *formation* of the self. So have also significant people around the subject. The subject has, through exercise and training, acquired a set of capacities and skills. The subject has with the help of others reached a level of autonomy. And he or she has entered and been included in one or more communities. Thus the self, which is the ground for the dignity of identity, has in a sense been partly *created* by the subject. But fundamental parts of the self are given by nature; the basic physical and mental dispositions and the looks of the person are given, although they may indeed be improved and cared for by the subject.

Could one not say, however, that the subjects attribute dignity to themselves through their evaluation of the self? To this my answer is that evaluation cannot by itself count as attribution of dignity. Much evaluation, for instance in the case of dignity of merit, presupposes that dignity is already there.

Against these observations the following argument can be raised. The attribution of dignity occurs on another level than that of the individual. The individual in many cases creates or achieves a state of affairs that constitutes the *ground* for a state of dignity. But dignity is not identical with its ground. I have said that dignity is a position on a value scale. The value scale is something created by humans and, it may be argued, is applied to various individuals and in that sense attributed to them. Instead of saying that dignity is attributed to the individual we now move to the idea of saying that the dignity scale has been attributed to human beings or to a particular community.

Again this is a quite plausible idea when it comes to some of the dignities of merit. In sports and in the scientific world there are competitions to be won and other targets to be reached in order for the individual to acquire the status of, for example, a world champion or a doctor. Sometimes such achievements are accompanied by nominations or appointments, but sometimes they are not. Achieving the level itself counts as reaching a dignity according to a scale previously created by society.

There may be other much more vague scales of merit, in a sense negotiated by members of society for assessing achievements, where one could argue in a similar way. But what about the dignities of moral stature and identity? In the case of morals we enter the profound problem of the nature and foundation of morals. I cannot tackle this problem here. Suffice it to say that by no means all schools of ethics regard morality as a convention or as a result of negotiation between people, and Sulmasy as a Catholic would clearly not do so. If the criteria of morality have been attributed to humans at all, the source, according to Christians, is God. But this must also be the case for human dignity which, according to Sulmasy, is an intrinsic property.

Dignity of identity is even more difficult. It is hard to disentangle what are attributions and what are not. I can only sketch an analysis here. There is in a society a general idea about what people should be like, what capacities, what freedom they should have and what they should minimally achieve in life. This idea is to a great extent culturally formed. Thus, this value scale is in a sense preformed. Individuals often judge themselves according to such a value scale, or are at least influenced by such a scale, when, for instance, they assess that dignity is lost. (See Edgar 2004 for an interesting analysis of the possible grounds for dignity.)

But some people are quite original and do not follow the common norms. They form their own identities and they assess their personal dignity according to a scale different from a conventional one. They may think that they have lost some of their identity when they have lost some very specific ability that not all other people would consider important. A poet would say that she has lost her dignity when she can no longer write poems. A diver would say that he has lost his dignity when he can no longer dive.

It is tempting to say here that the poet has produced her own scale of values or has attributed it to herself. But again, as in the case of morality, the poet need not – and we as analysts need not – look upon it that way. Evaluation is not tantamount to attributing a value scale to something. One may take the value scale as given, objectively given or otherwise intuitively understood, and evaluate according to it.

The dichotomy between intrinsic and attributed types of dignity is not, as I think I have shown, automatically helpful. This is not to deny the profound difference between human dignity and other types of dignity. The former is tied to human nature in general, it is equal in all humans and it exists as long as the person lives. The latter are tied to special properties or achievements of the individual; they differ between humans and they may come and go. Can we find new terms for the dichotomy? Here are two suggestions: *intrinsic and temporary* kinds of dignity and *unshakeable and vulnerable* kinds of dignity.

2.4.2 A critique of the four-notion typology

The four-notion typology of dignity analysed above (and first presented in Nordenfelt 2004) has been challenged in certain respects in an article by Wainwright & Gallagher (2008). These authors question the place and importance of this typology in the care of older people. I will here briefly address their critical points.

Wainwright and Gallagher doubt that all four types can 'form the basis of human worth'. They find, in particular, that the category of dignity of merit is irrelevant for the context of care. They also find my characterisation of the dignity of identity to be insufficient. It seems fatal, they think, to tie the dignity of identity so closely to the integrity and autonomy of the person. Individuals can maintain self-respect and dignity of identity even when their integrity or autonomy has been violated.

Space prevents me from commenting on details in this criticism. I wish however here to make a few statements in order to avoid certain misunderstandings. First, although I present this kind of typology in the context of the care of older people, my principal aim has been to make a basic and general analysis of the concept(s) of dignity. The fact that I mention the four types of dignity in parallel with each other does not mean that I find them all to be equally relevant in health care or the care of older people. It is clear from my presentations that human dignity and dignity of identity are the two types that are most relevant in the context of care. The dignity of moral stature is also relevant, but in a different way from the others. We should not require a particular moral status from the object of care, i.e. the patient or the client, in order to provide adequate care. We should, however, require a high moral status from the provider of the care. The provider should act morally, i.e. in a dignified way. Second, my idea in providing this list is not to say that these kinds of dignity can be added to each other in order to sustain the idea of human value in general. Instead, as I see it, they represent quite different kinds of value that are not additive. The most important value is the basic human dignity or *Menschenwürde*, and that is what we normally call the specifically human value. Third, the critics are quite right in observing that there are relationships between the items in my typology. To trace these relationships is a project worth pursuing and I have myself initiated such an enterprise in this book. I have here in particular compared human dignity and dignity of identity and noted resemblances and differences.

My fourth and final comment is related to an interesting observation by Wainwright and Gallagher. They are sceptical about my way of connecting dignity of identity to integrity and autonomy. They say that an older person may very well become distorted by illness and other bodily changes. Their autonomy may have become diminished. Still, the person may have retained their self-respect and may therefore, they claim, have retained a high degree of dignity of identity.

A full reply to this crucial observation requires much space and much reflection. I will now just make some preliminary observations. First, the comment by Wainwright and Gallagher points to the difficult relationship between a person's self-respect (or self-image) and their dignity of identity. As Wainwright and Gallagher claim, one person with a violated integrity can retain self-respect and a strong self-image whereas another person with an equally violated integrity can be shattered and feel that they have 'lost their dignity'. But does it follow from this that their dignities of identity are different?

According to my understanding, self-respect or self-image influences dignity of identity but does not completely determine it. (See my analysis of dignity of identity above.) If it did, we would have to draw some counter-intuitive conclusions. Assume that a boy with learning difficulties is grossly humiliated by another person who keeps ridiculing him in front of others. The boy, however, does not understand the insolence. He does not feel disturbed or feel that his integrity has been violated. On the other hand, many bystanders are deeply disturbed and they would, I claim, rightly insist that the person's integrity has been violated and that his dignity of identity has been reduced.

Thus although I see the force of Wainwright and Gallagher's observation it need not undermine my basic understanding of the concept of dignity of identity.

2.5 *Dignity and older people*

When I was a child I used to respect older people, but I don't notice that any more. For instance when you travelled by tram and an older person boarded the tram … you gave up your seat.

That doesn't happen today, you keep your seat (65-year-old Swedish man, Dignity and Older Europeans/Young and Middle-aged People, p. 30).

Let me now turn to the more specific question of whether there is a special dignity attached to older people. Is there such a dignity, or why should we otherwise pay special attention to older people? Or, do any of the mentioned varieties of dignity apply more significantly to older people?

Let us first consider human dignity as the basic starting point. Every older person has an intrinsic basic value, which entails a number of rights, among others the rights of the UN Declaration. The older person does not lose any of these rights because of reaching a particular age. It is a different matter that a few of the rights do not apply to older people because of their age, for instance the right to proper school education or the right to work. But this does not distinguish older people from infants. Other basic rights, on the other hand, have greater relevance to older people, for instance the universal right to care in the case of illness or disability.

Human dignity covers a great deal of ground when it comes to respecting the dignity of older people. Indeed, in spite of its basic position in all our human philosophies, this value is worth emphasising, since it is in practice so often violated, not least in institutions for older people. A reason behind such violation may be the relatively low public status that older people have in many circles, in particular among the very young. Human dignity does not, however, cover the whole ground of dignity relevant to older people. I want to explore to some extent the idea that older people may have certain specific dignities of merit.

First of all, many older people have personal dignities of merit. They may be aristocrats, high government officials, academics or artists. Others have struggled extremely hard in their professions or in their various walks of life, and deserve a merit of the 'Mother Teresa' kind. This may also have some, but rather limited, importance when these people grow old. When an official is no longer an official, it is rarely proper to pay attention to their former privileges or rights as an official. Moreover, many older people cannot rely on such a record. They may not have not been fortunate enough or they have not had the opportunity or the wish to earn merit in any particular respect.

Still, is there not something that is unique to all older people? They have all lived a long life and they have much experience of the various hardships and blessings in life. They know what life is all about. All this is a necessary part, but probably not the whole, of the crucial virtue of *wisdom*. My conjecture then is that all older people have the dignity of merit of wisdom.

The conjecture is not original. For some cultures – particularly prominent examples are the cultures of China and Japan – this assumption is a cornerstone. On the basis of the ancient Confucian teachings, older people have always been treated with much reverence and care in these countries. (For a thorough analysis of the Chinese situation, see for instance Engelhardt 2007.)

Although I think that we should share this Confucian attitude to older people, I realise that I must back up my position with much more argument. As I indicated above, a long life's experience, with all its necessary ingredients of education, work, love, frustrated love, disappointments, bereavement, illness, but also quite often of blessings of partnership and children, provides a good basis for wisdom, to many people a sufficient basis. But I believe some gift is required – although not a remarkable one – to digest these experiences properly, so that wisdom develops. We know that some people do not have even this minimal gift and we sometimes say of them that 'They will never learn'.

But what is wisdom, then? It is a kind of knowledge; it is not, however, just the simple knowledge of a fact, or even the complicated knowledge of a scientific system. Wisdom is knowledge whose object is life, more specifically human life. The wise person knows what life is like in general. The wise person also understands the complications of life. But wisdom is also practical knowledge in the sense that wise people know what to do in a particular situation, mainly because they have already experienced a similar situation before (cf. Aristotle's notion of *phronesis*, which entails the skill to apply ethical principles to individual cases). The wise person must to some extent be a moral person. I doubt, however, that we should identify wisdom with morality. I trace a fascinating element in wisdom that is such that wise people may sometimes challenge morality, at least traditional morality.

Let this suffice as a preliminary analysis. It seems clear that not everyone can attain wisdom, even if they have experienced a great deal in life. Some people may be apt to forget, and some people may lack the minimal intelligence necessary for wisdom. Moreover, even if we accept that all older people are wise in some way, they must be wise to different degrees. Some older people have experienced more variety in life; a few have experienced extreme horrors, whereas others have lived an extremely uniform and sheltered life. Some older people have more intellectual and emotional gifts than others. This means that some older people have had more ability to learn from life than others and thus their wisdom cannot be equal.

So if wisdom is a virtue particularly pertaining to older people, and constituting the special dignity of merit of older people, then there is a variation among older people with regard to this dignity. Is this a reason for treating older people differently? There may be reasons for doing so in certain respects. I think we should pay respect to the wise, particularly in the sense that we ought to listen to them on many occasions and often follow their advice. But there is no reason to treat the wise differently from the unwise when it comes to basic rights or to priority-setting with regard to basic goods. On this level the equal human dignity operates.

Although the idea of wisdom cannot be accepted immediately, it might be on the right track for establishing a common dignity of merit for older people. For this I wish to argue with the help of one line of argument used for the basic human dignity.

The normally cited grounds for human dignity are that humans have reason and self-consciousness, the ability to act freely, and the ability to set their own norms (autonomy). These endowments are probably peculiar to human beings; at least this seems to hold for autonomy. Only humans seem to be able to reflect on themselves in the sense that they can see alternative modes of conduct and choose what they consider to be the right rules for their conduct.

However, when human dignity has been contested in debate it has been noted that different individuals have these capacities to a different extent. Some are more rational than others; some can act more freely than others, the mentally well can act more freely than the mentally ill; the rich can act more freely than the poor; and some have a greater ability to set norms and indeed be conscious of norms. Moreover, there are examples of humans who have these gifts to a lesser extent than some higher animals. But if reason, free action and autonomy are the grounds for human dignity, then it seems to follow that different humans have different degrees of human dignity.

This reasoning is highly disturbing for the secular notion of human dignity. The Christian notion, on the other hand, is not affected. The idea of the human being as being in the image of God is quite different. According to Christian reasoning all humans, including psychopaths and people who are mentally ill, have been created in the image of God. But how can we save consistent reasoning in the case of the secular version of human dignity? One possible way is to give it up and say that there is no common equal human value. Such a conclusion would, however, have dramatic consequences for our civilisation. People would then, in the name of ethics, be treated differently and in accordance with their different endowments. This would also greatly influence the basis of the democratic political system.

Few of us could even consider living in such a society. For one thing, it would be tremendously complicated; we would need the most onerous bureaucracy to calculate people's gifts and put them on the right rung of the *Menschenwürde* ladder. One might wonder whether we could live in such a society, which would almost certainly foster cruelty and unhappiness as a consequence of some people feeling fundamentally superior and some fundamentally inferior.

Is there then another way of using the classical triad of reason, free action and autonomy for sustaining human dignity? One way of doing so is to lift the argument from the level of the individual to the level of the species. What is significant about the human species is, one might argue, that its individuals on the whole possess a degree of reason, capacity for free action and autonomy. On this basis, this species has a special high value. This high value is then also conferred on all individuals of this species, even if not all of them exemplify the grounds of the value. (For an interesting argument along these lines, see Sulmasy 2006.)

One could argue analogously with regard to older people and with regard to the special reason for revering older people. I have argued that not all older people are wise; therefore one cannot say that older people in general ought to be regarded as wise and treated in accordance with such a judgement. The idea now, however, is that it is typical for older people to be wiser than younger people because of their long experience of life. Thus it is a *typical* virtue of older people to be wise. Hence wisdom is a dignity of merit that could be ascribed to older people as a group, although not all older individuals exhibit wisdom. Thus, by analogy with human dignity that attaches to all humans regardless of their individual capacities, wisdom could be ascribed to all older people, regardless of their individual abilities and achievements in this respect.

But we may add a further argument for paying particular reverence to older people. That reason is *gratitude*. We normally owe a debt of gratitude to our older people. This is particularly so within the family. Children have a lot to thank their parents for. Parents have cared for and brought up their children for perhaps 20 years; they have put in an enormous amount of work. The financial support parents provide is often substantial; their care and love are often unlimited. Paradoxically, however, in today's Western culture this is less and less recognised. Parental care is taken for granted, even shrugged off. It is rare that young people recognise their deep debt to their parents. The due recognition of parents' love and effort has largely become restricted to religious practice. It is time for secular society to wake up to it.

Gratitude does not only have a place within the family. As young citizens we ought to thank our forefathers for their achievements in building up modern society, for their struggles in defence of democracy and other values, and in general for their intensive labour in keeping society working. Gratitude, I therefore suggest, is an appropriate attitude that we should display towards older people. Gratitude is our way of paying respect to a special dignity of merit that older people have. Let me call it the *dignity of achievement and effort*. This merit is a result of a wide variety of achievements and efforts on the part of older people for the good of humanity.

This, of course, does not mean that there are no young people who deserve gratitude more than some older ones. What is crucial in this context is that the proper time to show gratitude in some deeper and more general sense is when the person deserving gratitude has reached a certain age. Compare this with the way we pay a particular tribute to a person who is retiring or leaving a job for some other reason. We then sum up all the person's achievements and efforts and thank them for all they have done. In a similar way older people are approaching the end of their life, so it is timely to make a summing up and show some general gratitude for it all.

But is it reasonable to say that we should be as grateful to elderly train robbers as to Mother Teresa? Obviously not: there must always be a case for specific and adequate gratitude for specific deeds or, in the case of Mother Teresa, for lifelong outstanding achievements. What I am arguing for is a basic general attitude of gratitude towards all older people. Nearly all of them have done a lot of good and worked very hard. My point is that we should assume that this is so in our attitude towards all of them and act accordingly. In terms of wisdom, most older people have something important to say or show us about life. We ought to presume that this is the case for every older person we meet, and pay due reverence. This does not preclude paying particular attention and respect to the really wise.

There is one further important reason for treating older people with special consideration, but it is not a dignity of older people; rather, it relates to their special *vulnerability*. By this I mean both physical vulnerability, the fact that older people are more disposed to injury and disease than others, and their existential vulnerability. Older people are approaching the end of their lives. Their *Angst* (to use the term made current by the German philosopher Martin Heidegger) or mental suffering becomes more pronounced. They may not have prepared themselves at all for the idea of death, a thought that may suddenly dawn upon them, often in conjunction with some illness. For them, death may be an imminent reality. And what does that mean to them? How can older people find a motive for continuing to live and doing so in a harmonious way? As younger people, we have a special responsibility for supporting our older brothers and sisters in this regard. (This section summarises my account in Nordenfelt 2003. For interesting comparisons with my discussion about dignity and older people, see Moody 1998 and Agich 2007.)

Box 2.1   The art of identifying the species of dignity

Here I exemplify the various species of dignity by considering some particular cases and indicating how the various types of dignity can be identified.

Easy cases
In these cases the type of dignity is made explicit.

Dignity is a value attached to all human beings to the same extent (human dignity, *Menschenwürde*).

Some patients do not respect the dignity of doctors (dignity of merit).

The nurse acted in a really dignified way towards the dying woman (dignity of moral stature).

I lost my dignity when my leg was amputated (dignity of identity).

Overlapping cases
The situation becomes a bit more complicated when two kinds of dignity are involved at the same time. This frequently holds for dignity of human dignity and dignity of identity.

This man's dignity was violated when he was kidnapped.

Here there is an infringement of the man's basic human right to live as a free person who can decide for himself. At the same time his identity is shattered, in terms of both autonomy and integrity. This overlap follows from the simple fact that some of the basic rights of an individual's human dignity concern the integrity and autonomy of this person.

Ambiguous cases
In these cases a sentence involving dignity can be interpreted in at least two ways.

You preserve the dignity of a person when you make her feel that she is of value.

This is an extremely general statement because of the unspecified word 'value'. The speaker could in fact be referring to most kinds of dignity: he may refer to the woman's merits, for instance her social position; to her moral stature; or to the particular value of her being the unique person she is.

Contextual cases

His contentment is a sign that dignity is there.

This statement of course also needs a lot of interpretation. But this interpretation does not only concern the kind of dignity referred to. We may here assume that the dignity referred to is dignity of identity. But a further fundamental question concerns the relation between contentment and dignity. We have at least three possibilities:

- The contentment is a part of dignity.
- The contentment is an effect of dignity.
- The contentment is a cause of dignity.

All three interpretations seem plausible and thus the statement is in need of further explication. Although contentment cannot be a necessary condition of a specific case of dignity of identity, it can be an integral part of a person's self-esteem, for instance. Self-esteem is a part of a person's identity. Contentment can obviously be an effect of a person's awareness of the enhancement or preservation of their dignity of identity. Conversely, when a person is generally content with life their dignity be enhanced.

References

Agich, G. (2007) Reflections on the function of dignity in the context of caring for old people. *Journal of Medicine and Philosophy*, **32**, 483–494.

Birnbacher, D. (1996) Ambiguities in the concept of *Menschenwürde*. In: *Sanctity of Life and Human Dignity* (ed K. Bayertz), pp. 107–121, Kluwer, Dordrecht.

Collins English Dictionary (2003), 6th edn. HarperCollins, London.

Diccionario de la Lengua Española (2001), edited by Real Academia Española. Espasa, Madrid.

DOE (2004) Dignity and Older Europeans *Project Final Report of Focus Groups (2002–2004)*. http://www.cardiff.ac.uk/dignity.

Edgar, A. (2004) A response to Nordenfelt's 'The varieties of dignity'. *Health Care Analysis*, **12**, 83–89.

Engelhardt, H.T. Jr (2007) Long-term care: the family, post-modernity, and conflicting moral life-worlds. *Journal of Medicine and Philosophy*, **32**, 519–536.

Franklin, L.-L., Ternestedt, B.-M. & Nordenfelt, L. (2006) Views on dignity of elderly nursing home residents. *Nursing Ethics*, **13**, 1–15.

Honneth, A. (1992) Integrity and disrespect: principles of a conception of morality based on the theory of recognition. *Political Theory*, **20**, 187–201.

Kant, I. (1997) *Foundations of the Metaphysics of Morals*. Translated with an introduction by L.W. Beck. Prentice Hall, Upper Saddle River, NJ.

Kolnai, A. (1976) Dignity. *Philosophy*, **51**, 251–271.

Krátky slovník slovenského jazyka (2006), ed. K. Buzassoya & A. Jorosova. Veda, Bratislava.

Moody, H.R. (1998) Why dignity in old age matters. In: *Dignity and Old Age* (eds R. Disch, R. Dobrof & H.R. Moody), pp. 13–38. Haworth Press, New York.

MSN-Encarta Online Dictionary (2007) www.encarta.msn.com/encnet/features/dictionary.

Nationalencyklopedins ordbok (2004), ed. Språkdata, Gothenburg University. Bra Böcker, Höganäs.

Nordenfelt, L. (2003) Dignity and the care of the elderly. *Medicine, Health Care and Philosophy*, **6**, 103–110.

Nordenfelt, L. (2004) The varieties of dignity. *Health Care Analysis*, **12**, 69–81.

Nouveau petit Robert: dictionnaire alphabétique et analogique de la langue française (2007), ed. J. Rey-Debove, A. Rey, S. Chantreau & M.-H. Drivaud. Dictionnaires de Robert, Paris.

Oxford Dictionary of English (2007). Oxford University Press, Oxford.

Pico della Mirandola, G. (1948) On the dignity of man. In: *The Renaissance Philosophy of Man* (eds E. Cassirer, P.O. Kristeller & J.H. Randall), pp. 215–254. University of Chicago Press, Chicago.

Słownik Języka Polskiego (1978) [The Polish Language Dictionary], vol.1 (ed. M. Szymczak). PWN, Warszawa.

Spiegelberg, H. (1970) Human dignity: a challenge to contemporary philosophy. In: *Human Dignity: This Century and the Next* (eds R. Gotesky & E. Laszlo), pp. 39–64. Gordon & Breach, Amsterdam.

Statman, Z. (1986) Dignity and responsibility. *Dialectics and Humanism*, **Nos 2–3**, 193–205.

Statman, D. (2000) Humiliation, dignity and self-respect. *Philosophical Psychology*, **13**, 523–540.

Sulmasy, D.P. (1997) Death with dignity: what does it mean? *Josephinum Journal of Theology*, **4**, 13–23.

Sulmasy, D.P. (2006) Dignity and the human as a natural kind. In: *Health and Human Flourishing: Religion, Medicine and Moral Anthropology* (eds C.R. Taylor & R. Dell'Oro), pp. 71–87. Georgetown University Press, Washington DC.

United Nations (1948) *The Universal Declaration of Human Rights*, adopted and proclaimed by General Assembly resolution 217 A (111) of 10 December 1948. Office of the High Commissioner for Human Rights, Geneva.

Velký sociologický slovník (1996), ed. H. Marikova, M. Petrusek & A. Vodakova. Alena – Univerzita Karlova, Prague.

Wainwright, P. & Gallagher, A. (2008) On different types of dignity in nursing care: a critique of Nordenfelt. *Nursing Philosophy*, **9**, 46–54.

3. *Being Body: The Dignity of Human Embodiment*

Jennifer Bullington

Introduction

The human body is a remarkable phenomenon in the natural world. Our bodies are made up of material substances, such as skin and bones, muscles and nerve tissue, but they also 'contain' something non-material, something that has been called the soul, or psyche, self-consciousness or person, to use more modern terminology. However, the notion of the body-as-container of the soul is a problematic, dualistic way of describing a human being. The philosophical standpoint of dualism (mind–body split) has been riddled with problems since the time of Descartes. What is the nature of the relationship between the physical and the non-physical, between mind and body, between meaning and material? How is all this to be understood? Modern medicine has further cemented this notion of the body as a container or thing through the detailed study of the mechanical, material aspects of the body. This machine body, or 'objective' body, is the focus of medical science and practice. It is by opening up the body, dissecting corpses and removing the person (subjectivity) from the human body that we have gained the natural-scientific knowledge that has enabled us to cure and prevent many diseases and health problems. Our everyday notions about the body are formed by this natural-scientific view of the body. In the course of this chapter I will argue that this perspective, no matter how ingrained in our understanding, is in fact not the primary view of the body. Understanding the body in objectifying terms is a derived, constructed perspective on the body that we live at every moment. The body that we live at every moment is hidden from view because we have learned to regard the body as a thing.

In medical practice, the personal body of the patient is most often put aside in order to investigate the objective body. This means that the body that we *live* is not in focus in the traditional medical encounter. Furthermore, the experience of pain, injury and disease in itself alienates us from our own bodies, which we experience as obstinate, disturbing things that are in the way, like a broken machine. Thus, our everyday notions of our bodies as things, as well as the experience of pain and disease, lead to a certain way of viewing the body that ignores the most important aspect of the human body

54

– that is, it is *someone's* body. The objective body, described and investigated by medicine, represents only one way of viewing the body.

An alternative way of regarding the human body is to understand it as a *lived* body, i.e. as a mind–body unity in the world. In this way of thinking, our embodied presence in the world is the ground for all knowledge and experience. It is in and through our bodies that we exist and can have contact with and knowledge about the world. To understand the body in this way implies a radical change in perspective from the body as a thing. We do not *have* bodies, we *are* bodies, which gives the body a special status among worldly phenomena. The human body, or rather, the embodied human being, is the place where the world reveals itself, a nexus of meaning and signification that radiates from the human body towards things and other beings. Being embodied is being situated and oriented towards a field of experience as *this* body, *this* history, *this* psyche, *this* point of view. The dignity of the human body has to do with affirming the lived body as an expression of a unique perspective, as an opening upon the world, not to be confused with the objective body, understood as an anonymous collection of bones and tissue. In this chapter I explore this alternative to the notion of the body-container by examining the French phenomenologist Maurice Merleau-Ponty's (1945/1962) notion of the lived body. Furthermore, the special case of the ageing body will be discussed. The failing faculties and vulnerability of old age present a special challenge in modern societies that place the highest value on qualities such as competence, competition and productivity. Implications of this for health care and the care of older people will then be discussed.

This chapter will begin by making clear the distinction between the body-as-thing (third-person perspective) and the body-as-me (first-person perspective). Because of the ambiguity of the human body, as embodied consciousness, it is possible to entertain both these notions of the body, even though the body as 'it' or 'thing' is the most common way of conceptualising the body, in both lay and professional language. It is as if we lack words for the experience of *being* bodies. The objectivistic view of the human body stands in the way of discovering the lived body, understood as a mind–body unity in the world. We need to find words to describe the lived, non-thematic experience of the body-as-me.

In this chapter, the dignity of the lived body will be exemplified in relation to two themes: the body and knowledge and the body and self. The first theme will be illustrated through the work of writers from different traditions who all assert the vital role of the body for knowledge, reason and meaning. Since the time of Plato the body has been considered to be a source of error and deception, not to be trusted in the important task of ascertaining true knowledge. Over the centuries there has been an effort to keep bodies out of philosophy, science and other intellectual activities. However, as we shall see, there is good reason for calling this strategy into question. The philosophical anthropologist Maxine Sheets-Johnstone (1990, 1994), the linguist and philosopher Mark Johnson (1987) and the phenomenologist Hans Jonas (1966) provide arguments for including the body in the 'higher' functions such as cognition, imagination and reason. These authors are not referring to the objective body, conceptualised in natural-scientific terms (i.e. brain processes and hormones), but to the lived body, understood as the source and genesis of meaning. In the second theme, the relationship between the lived body and the self will be examined, and the case of the aged body will be discussed.

3.1   The objective body and the lived body

3.1.1   Objectivistic epistemology (theory of knowledge) and phenomenology

In order to clarify the terms 'objective body' and 'lived body' it is necessary first to examine the corresponding epistemological perspectives underlying these terms. I have already mentioned briefly the objectivistic point of view, a view that could be characterised as 'the view from nowhere' (Nagel 1989). This perspective could also be called a God's eye view, where it is assumed that there exists an independent reality that can be correctly described in symbolic representations (language) corresponding to things and relationships in the 'real world'. According to the objectivistic view there is a neutral perspective beyond human limitations and independent of human subjectivity and embodiment, a transcendent 'objective' stance outside of the person–world relationship, in which the alleged correspondence between things and what-is-said-about-things can be judged. Knowledge is objective, in the sense that it can be verified as factual states of affairs in the real world. The ideal of objectivity is one of the most prominent characteristics of natural science. The idea of a subject-independent reality is so ingrained in our cultural thinking that it is difficult to imagine knowledge and meaning in any other way. But however useful this perspective may be in other contexts, it prevents us from grasping the subjective elements in thinking and understanding. In order to grasp the subjective in a positive way, and not merely as a disturbing interfering variable, we need another way of thinking about knowledge and meaning. Phenomenology can reveal this dimension by the adoption of a stance other than the objectivistic one.

Phenomenology is a philosophical movement in European philosophy stemming from the works of Edmund Husserl (1913/1962, 1954/1970). The term means literally the *logos* (or inherent meaning or order) of phenomena, that is to say, the meaning of that which appears or shows itself to us. How human beings perceive, understand and live the world is the subject matter of phenomenological study. In other words, the realm of subjectivity is the focus of interest. Husserl's life project was to establish phenomenology as a rigorous science, on a par with the natural sciences that studied nature. However, since the subject matter for phenomenology differs in kind from the subject matter of the natural sciences, Husserl was forced to create a methodology and concepts that would be suitable for the study of human 'meaning constitution', to use another term. He understood that the objective methodologies, so successful in natural science, would not do justice to the subjective. The study of 'appearances' would need a new approach. This approach was worked out in Husserl's phenomenological thinking and gave inspiration to an entire phenomenological movement. (See Spiegelberg 1982 for a comprehensive overview of the phenomenological movement.)

Without going into detail, one can summarise the radical change in perspective from the objectivity of the natural sciences to the phenomenological study of subjectivity as a shift of focus. Instead of studying the world of objects in the material world, as the natural scientist does, phenomenologists, having decided to study another realm, had to place the 'real' objective world in brackets, the so-called *epoché*, or phenomenological reduction. The term 'reduction' by no means implies reducing wholes to parts or looking for the least common denominator. Reduction here means that the reality status of the world and the objective qualities of things are put into suspension in order to concentrate on an area that is non-thematic and impossible to see as long as the objective perspective is dominant.

By putting aside all interest in the existence of the real world and the objective qualities of things, phenomenology shifted focus to the manner of appearance, to the way in which human consciousness attends to that which appears. The focus of interest is how things present themselves (manner of presentation) and how consciousness 'constitutes' the meaning of that which appears. This constitution of meaning is discovered by examining the stream of consciousness towards that which is outside of consciousness. Within phenomenology the technical term for the stream of consciousness towards something outside itself is 'intentionality'. This is a term Husserl borrowed from Brentano (1982), characterising the way in which consciousness 'intends' its objects. In order to study the way in which consciousness intends or constitutes its object ('object' here referring to that towards which consciousness flows), the reality status of the world must be put aside. This does not mean that phenomenologists deny the existence of the real world, it merely announces another focus of interest, requiring its own methods and terminology. Working out this philosophical strategy was Husserl's life project.

A common misunderstanding about phenomenology is that the study of 'appearances' is less important than the study of the real world. An appearance is, after all, merely an appearance, less viable than real things, certainly secondary in importance to the study of real transcendent objects. We tend to give natural-scientific descriptions of things a higher status than the world we experience through our senses. However, Husserl (1954/1970) pointed out that the world we experience is in fact primordial, that is to say, prior to natural-scientific descriptions of the world. We saw round objects in the world before this experience became abstracted into the mathematical concept of the circle. We saw how grains of sand make up a continuous stretch of beach before we started to construct theories about particles and atoms. According to Husserl, it is precisely on the basis of lived experience (i.e. 'appearances') that we have been able to construct the abstract terminology and explanations conceptualised by natural science. Unfortunately, according to Husserl (1954/1970) we have forgotten this grounding of science in the experience of the world, and this forgetting has resulted in the deprecation of the so-called 'life-world' (*Lebenswelt*), the taken-for-granted everyday world of common experience. We find ourselves immersed in the life-world, consisting of values, beliefs, assumptions and cultural practices. The life-world is the unproblematic, pre-scientific world that constitutes the meaning of everyday life. Phenomenology affirms the life-world and the study of appearances as vital areas of study.

To reiterate, phenomenology does not make statements about how the world is in itself, outside of human beings' experiences of it. The subject matter of phenomenological studies is experiences of various human phenomena such as perception, time consciousness, sexuality, and religious and cultural expressions of meaning. In order to study these phenomena, it is necessary to implement the phenomenological reduction (bracket the reality character of the world) and focus upon the world-as-meant, or world-as-intended. When we do this, we find, according to Husserl, two poles of experience, one of which corresponds to the stream of consciousness (*noesis* or noetic acts) and the other of which corresponds to that which consciousness attends to (*noema* or noematic objects). In place of the objective 'real' object we find, under the phenomenological reduction, the stream of consciousness towards the object as meant. This bracketed realm of noesis and noema is the study of phenomenology proper.

It is beyond the scope of this chapter to give a detailed account of the phenomenological method. In this context it suffices to say that phenomenology is an alternative to objectivistic epistemology, an alternative that takes its starting point in how the world appears to human beings. The phenomenon that will be examined in this chapter is the experience of being body. The phenomenological perspective will be used in order to elucidate the phenomenon of human embodiment. In order to do this, I turn to the phenomenologist who has sometimes been called 'the philosopher of the body', Maurice Merleau-Ponty.

3.1.2 Merleau-Ponty's phenomenology

Merleau-Ponty had a good idea of what he wanted to accomplish even as a young doctoral student. At the age of 25 he submitted two research proposals that contained the themes he would come to work with in his first two philosophical texts, *The Structure of Behavior* (1942) and *Phenomenology of Perception* (1945). The focus of these two works was a phenomenological reflection on the nature of perception and human embodiment. Later in his career he turned his attention to a variety of other topics, such as language acquisition (1964/1973), expression and meaning (1960/1964) and literature and art (1948/1964; 1969/1973), but his interest in perception and the body remained with him throughout his career. His last work, *The Visible and the Invisible*, published posthumously in 1964 from his working notes, showed how he had returned to the theme of the embodied human being and the world. The concept 'flesh of the world' used in this last work was meant to describe the event where perception and meaning are born, not as a relationship between a constituting subject and a constituted object but as an intertwining or ensemble of being. He questioned the privileged position given to consciousness within phenomenology and maintained that we need to find another way to investigate the human world. We do not need to follow his thoughts as far as this, but it is interesting to see how he spent his entire philosophical career reflecting on the embodiment of nature and how embodied human beings experience the world.

Merleau-Ponty shows how many of our ideas about the human body and the nature of perception are conditioned by notions and concepts from natural science. These notions make it hard for us to reflect upon and discover how we experience our bodies in the world, and how we experience the world through our bodies. We understand perception, for example, in terms of stimulus–response. Although we never experience a stimulus as such, we are convinced that perception is 'really' all about light waves hitting the occipital lobe in the brain. This is, of course, a perfectly legitimate way of describing perception from a certain perspective, but it is not the way we live perception. If we focus only on chemical, neurological processes, we miss the way in which the experience and meaning of the world unfolds for us. Human experience is the result of a unique relation between the embodied subject and that which shows itself to us at every instant. The subject and the world are 'born together' (the word for knowledge in French is *connaissance*, which means literally, born together) in a movement that has been poorly understood by both science and philosophy. We need to bracket our everyday notions about the objective body and natural-scientific notions about the nature of perception in order to elucidate the 'dialogue' between the subject and their world.

How then to disclose this uncharted territory? Merleau-Ponty begins by assuring us that there is certainly something outside ourselves that we are born into, which we have no choice but to relate to in one way or another. This 'something' is present to us in ways that we experience through our senses. But this world outside ourselves is not imprinted upon us like a photograph, but taken up in a moment of active constitution of meaning. Merleau-Ponty (1945/1962) describes this meeting in the following way:

> Thus a sensible datum which is on the point of being felt sets a kind of muddled problem for my body to solve. I must find the attitude which *will* provide it with the means of becoming determinate, of showing up as blue; I must reply to a question which is obscurely expressed. And yet I do so only when I am invited by it, my attitude is never sufficient to make me really see blue or really touch a hard surface … As I contemplate the blue of the sky I am not over and against it as an acosmic subject; I do not possess it in thought, or spread out towards it some idea of blue such as might reveal the secret of it, I abandon myself to it and plunge into this mystery, it 'thinks itself within me' … (p. 214, italics in original).

> Apart from the probing of my eye or my hand, and before my body synchronizes with it, the sensible is nothing but a vague beckoning (p. 214).

The classical subject–object dichotomy is loosened up and we find an area 'between' subject and object, and it is only within this area that the experience of what we call the world can arise. To take an illustrative example, imagine the figure–ground phenomenon, a well-known principle from gestalt psychology. I may look out of the window to see if my friend has arrived, or I may change perspective and notice that the window is dirty and needs to be cleaned. Both of these perspectives are possible, but they are not 'in' the view in any objective way. Foreground and background only exist between a subject who meets a view with certain interests and attention, and a world that shows itself in terms of the subject's interests and attention. We cannot see both the smudge on the window and the friend coming up the drive at the same time, as illustrated by the famous perceptual example, taken from gestalt psychology, of the vase and the two faces (see Figure 3.1). One can only see the vase or the faces, never both at the same time. Both are there simultaneously in the picture (objectively), but only available perceptually (subjectively) one at a time.

What is present perceptually thus depends on the subject. However, the subject needs to be given the opportunity to orient either towards the dirty window or the friend. One sees only what one is 'invited' to see, as Merleau-Ponty expresses it.

Figure–ground is a striking example of something that is constitutive of perception itself, that there is always a given perspective (interest, or 'meaning constitution') since there is always an embodied subject. Our mistake has been to lose sight of this relationship and divide up experience in terms of an objective world, understood in terms of natural science, and an objective, anonymous body that processes various stimuli in the brain. But the world is not an objective collection of things lying about, and the human body is not a processing machine. Again, this description is entirely correct if we wish to study the world from an objectivistic point of view, but here the interest is in phenomenology and the study of the subjective, so we put aside this naturalistic conceptualisation and examine experience in terms of subjectivity, embodiment and meaning

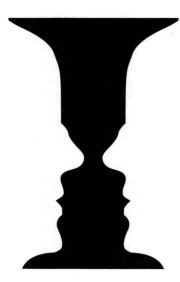

Figure 3.1 Figure–ground phenomenon.

constitution. If we disregard the subject–object dichotomy and focus upon the realm of the 'in-between', we will discover a lived unity that we could call a mind–body unity always present to the world, in one way or another. The 'world', again, being understood as the dialogue between the embodied human being and the presentation of something which beckons to us as an invitation to understand. Merleau-Ponty (1945/1962) writes, 'Inside and outside are inseparable. The world is wholly inside and I am wholly outside of myself' (p. 407) and 'The world is not what I think, but what I live through. I am open to the world, I have no doubt that I am in communication with it, but I do not possess it; it is inexhaustible' (pp. xvi–xvii).

3.1.3 The lived body
Merleau-Ponty calls the lived unity of the mind–body–world system the 'lived body'. The body understood as a lived body is necessarily ambiguous, since it is both material and self-conscious. It is physiological and psychological, but Merleau-Ponty asserts that these terms are not as dichotomous as one would imagine. There is mind in the body and body in the mind. Merleau-Ponty (1945/1962) again:

> Man taken as a concrete being is not a psyche joined to an organism, but the movement to and fro of existence which at one time allows itself to take corporeal form and at others moves towards personal acts. Psychological motives and bodily occasions may overlap because there is not a single impulse in a living body which is entirely fortuitous in relation to psychic intentions, not a single mental act which has not found at least its germ or its general outline in physiological tendencies (p. 88).

These realms are rather to be understood as levels, intertwined, constituting a unified field. The self, the body and the world of things and others are neither separated from each other nor to be confused with each other, but rather can be seen as three sectors or levels of a unique field. The lived body is always oriented towards the world outside itself (otherness) in a constant flow. The human being can be said to move on various levels on a mind–body continuum, depending upon the nature of the concrete situation. When needed, the level of mind comes to the fore and the physical level recedes into background. One does not cease to have a body in such situations, nor even cease to have bodily experiences, but these are placed at the margins of the field as the mental rises to meet the situation at hand. Giving a lecture or being interviewed on television or questioned by the police are situations that naturally call forth the reflective, cognitive level of the lived body. Likewise, when dancing, having a massage, floating on a raft in a pool or falling asleep, we let the psychological level of the field recede. If one were to be mostly 'body' at the police station, there would be a disharmony in the field. The situation would break down, the police would give up trying to ask questions and one would most probably be referred to a psychiatrist. By the same token, if one thinks too much, it will be impossible to dance, fall asleep or enjoy floating in the pool. The harmony-of-situation is based upon the smooth correspondence between the embodied subject and the meaning of the situation. One may, of course, misunderstand a situation, but this only occurs in cases where the ambiguity or newness of the situation does not provide any clues as to what one is experiencing. The harmony of the mind–body–world system is the norm; disharmony and ambiguity are exceptions.

The harmony of situations is 'sedimented', to use Merleau-Ponty's language, in terms of so-called 'structures', which allow the world to be apprehended in a rudimentary organisation which we already understand. Merleau-Ponty borrowed the idea of structure from gestalt psychology, although he gave the term a meaning beyond the gestalt psychologists' use of it. His development of the concept was to see structure as an 'in-between' phenomenon, neither in things nor in subjects but created in the meeting of the two. Structures are the bodily, psychological and social ways of being oriented towards the world that guide our understanding and through sedimentation give us freedom by presenting the world as familiar and known. Sedimented structures allow us to experience the world as comprehensible and manageable. We develop stable patterns of experience that tell us how to move our bodies, how to respond to various psychological and social situations, and how to understand our everyday ordinary life-world. These structures, built up over time, free our attention from having to form the 'base' of experience over and over again. Our maternal language and bodily repertoire are second nature to us: we do not have to re-learn them in every new situation. Such sedimentations are the necessary precondition for us to be able to communicate fluently and move about in an unencumbered way. The experience of learning a new language or a new motor skill makes us aware of how effortlessly these sedimented structures actually work. To have to think about which verb form to use or where to put the negation in a sentence shows us what language is like when it is not part of a sedimented structure. However, if we learn the new language well enough and use it for long enough, we may reach the point where even the second language becomes a part of our sedimented language repertoire. In such a case, we have acquired a new language structure. The ability to learn a new language illustrates the second important

61

aspect of structures; namely, that they are not only sedimented but also spontaneous. This means that we can develop our structures to fit new situations and challenges. Structures are thus both sedimented (organised into relatively fixed patterns) and spontaneous (capable of transformation), since the nature of the 'in-between' is to be in a constant flow of relation to ever-changing concrete situations.

The way in which structures are formed, change and develop can be illustrated by the experience of learning to drive a car. Before one learns to drive, the car is experienced merely as a means of transportation, or perhaps as a source of aesthetic pleasure. The 'car-structure' is not articulated in a nuanced way, but generalised, with little detail. Perceptually, I attend to the car door, the seat, perhaps the smell of the car and the sound of the engine, but over and above these blunt impressions nothing particular stands out. Bodily, the car-structure of the non-driver has to do with the way one moves one's body to get to the car, the feeling of the seat (on the passenger side), the passing view from the window. Before one can drive, the experience of the car will be at this level of articulation. However, all of this changes as soon as I place myself in the driver's seat and start to learn to drive. Firstly, my body will no longer be passively 'seated' in the car seat, but must become actively attuned to the pedals, gear shift, mirrors and steering wheel. The view from the window that was so entertaining and free from demands as a passenger suddenly becomes filled with questions (Which lane should I be in? When should I signal? Should I pass this car?) and demands (he is waiting for me to turn, I seem to be blocking traffic, I just missed a chance to enter the roundabout, they keep passing me, I'm probably driving too slowly, everyone is honking at me). When as the driver I listen to the engine, the sound is no longer experienced as the background noise of 'starting the car' but rather a noise to be queried: How does the engine sound? Is everything all right? In the first phases of learning to drive, I will have to filter every perception and motor activity through cognition, as there is as yet no sedimented structure for this experience. I will be hyper-present to my own body, to the functions of the car and the traffic in a way that experienced drivers have long forgotten. The passage from novice to experienced driver is accomplished when I 'have' the road and the car in my body. The driving becomes a harmonious field of experience where I move with ease. I am no longer hyper-aware of myself driving, nor in need of constant cognition in order to navigate the car in traffic. I can even lose myself in thought and not realise how I suddenly arrived home. There have even been reported incidences of people driving in their sleep as a side-effect of a certain type of sleeping medication. To an inexperienced driver, this sounds like an impossible feat.

The phenomenologist Kay Toombs (2001) describes the way her life-world became disrupted by the progressive disease muscular sclerosis. Things she used to do without thinking, like climbing the steps up to her classroom, became impossible, and situations that she previously mastered without a thought became complicated problems to solve. A swinging door, trying to put tights on immobile legs or eating a bowl of soup demanded the development of new strategic ways of relating to objects. This process is by no means easy. She writes:

> The surrounding world appears (feels) different than it did prior to bodily dysfunction. In particular, the world is experienced as overtly obstructive, surprisingly

non-accommodating. Actions are sensed as effortful, where hitherto they had been effortless. … When ceaseless and ongoing effort is required to perform the simplest of tasks (getting out of bed, dressing, taking a shower, going on a trip), there is a powerful impulse to withdraw, to cease doing what is required. The person with a disability is tempted severely to curtail involvements in the world (2001, p. 253).

The habitual way of moving and perceiving no longer 'works' in these challenging situations. Learning to adapt to chronic illness and disability means learning to inhabit a new world. Transforming our ways of seeing, moving and even feeling and thinking are all a part of what it means to 'cope' with challenging situations. And when we have transformed our structures, the world is not the same. Toombs again:

I catch myself watching students running across the campus, or colleagues taking the stairs two-at-a-time, and I marvel at their effortless ability to do so. Try as I might, I can no longer remember how it was to move like that. It is not simply that I cannot recall the last occasion when I walked upright. It is that I cannot recollect, or re-imagine, the felt bodily sense of 'walking' (2001, p. 254).

The above examples illustrate a process of structure transformation that is perpetually ongoing, even when we are not in an explicit process of learning a new skill or coping with a traumatic life change. We rely on sedimented structures for our grounding in a world that we already understand, yet we continually develop and transform our structures in line with the unfolding of situations. Through the process of living we are continually confronted with situations that challenge our sedimented structures and we are called upon to modify our bodily, psychological and social ways of being in the world. A tension arises in the field that calls for a new understanding, a revision of previous notions, or a new bodily pattern or motor activity. For example, one becomes paralysed and has to experience the world from a wheelchair, or one finds out that a lifelong friend has been sleeping with one's partner for years. Feelings, thoughts, memories and bodily experiences are challenged in such situations. The world is 'not the same' after such events. Even the normal process of ageing often gives rise to situations that challenge our taken-for-granted, everyday structures. The body breaks down, working life comes to an end, friends die. The lived body of age involves a variety of challenges that will be discussed in the final section of the chapter.

Merleau-Ponty's notion of the lived body and structure transformation provides a philosophical alternative to the objectivistic epistemology that focuses on the objective body, as seen from a God's eye perspective. The lived body is understood as a mind–body presence always directed towards the world (otherness). Therein arises a field, an 'in-between', that is constituted in terms of situations to be mastered and understood. From this perspective, the body plays a larger role in our experience than we are used to imagining. When we shift our focus from the objective body to the lived body, we discover a new area to explore.

I will now turn to exploring the body's integral role in areas of life that have not been traditionally associated with embodiment. The body, far from being an 'it', is in fact a vital dimension of the human being.

3.2   *The dignity of the human body*

The purpose of this section is to demonstrate how the body plays an integral part in our understanding of the world and can even be seen as constituting the ground of what we call our 'selves'. The dignity of the human body will be highlighted by examining the role of the body in knowledge acquisition and the body in relation to the self.

3.2.1   The body and knowledge

Although perception and knowledge are intimately connected, within Western philosophy and science we find a deep-seated suspicion of the body as a source of true knowledge. The senses are considered to be unreliable. It is argued that we are often deceived by what we see and hear, and we need to rely upon logic and rational thinking in order to acquire true knowledge about the world. The roots of this pessimism go all the way back to the ancient Greek philosopher Plato. In the Platonic dialogue *Theaetetus* (Plato 1961) we find Socrates in a discussion about the nature of knowledge. What is knowledge, and how do we attain it? A famous Sophist of the time, Protagoros, had claimed that 'man is the measure of all things'. Socrates argues against this premise by showing that it would imply that what things seem to be *for me* is how things actually are. If I see a cat over there, then there *is* a cat over there. But, as Socrates points out, it may very well be a large rat, or a shadow or a variety of other things. My thinking that I see a cat by no means enables me to say with absolute certainty that there actually is a cat over there. Not only can we be deceived by our senses, we may also end up in impossible intersubjective difficulties: for example, if you think it is cold outside and I think it is warm, is it actually warm or cold? There is no way to decide the issue if we simply rely on our subjective experiences. We will need some form of 'objective' point of view to solve the problem. Socrates had a solution that would not satisfy us today, referring to the world of ideas. But his critique of perception as a source of knowledge has stayed with us up to modern times. Science and philosophy have been guided by the notion that knowledge should be based upon objective criteria that effectively remove all the subjective elements of perception that tend to lead us astray. In this way, the body and perception have been banned from epistemology. However, we cannot ignore the fact that it is in and through our bodies and our perceptions that we have contact with the world. Regardless of which culture we come from or during which historical period of time we live, we experience the world through our bodies. It is in and through our bodies that we can have any kind of knowledge at all.

Let us now examine some authors who emphasise the role of the body in the 'higher' functions of cognition and meaning constitution. The philosophical anthropologist Maxine Sheets-Johnstone (1994) recounts that archaeologists and anthropologists have noted that the first tools human beings made seemed to perform the same work as teeth. Primitive hammers were constructed that pulverised material in the same way as the larger back teeth ground food, while the first wedge used to divide material in a precise manner could be seen as performing the same function as the thinner front teeth. Sheets-Johnstone argues that the first human tools could be said to be an externalisation of teeth. How did this transformation come about? According to Sheets-Johnstone we can understand the process in terms of a development from a bodily tactile experience, i.e.

the feeling of using teeth and the way teeth feel in the mouth, to a visual experience involving making a stone *look* the way the teeth *feel.* An evolutionary step forward occurred when the human being could *see* the line of the front teeth that she felt when drawing her tongue across them. This process of transformation from body experiences to visual externalisation became more sophisticated over time and eventually gave rise to more complex tools, buildings and finally the entire complex of psychological, cultural reality.

Sheets-Johnstone takes the eyes as offering a further example of how the body is involved in meaning constitution. In this case, body experiences of vision are transformed into abstract notions of interiority, otherness and holiness, concepts that we do not normally identify with the body. She begins her analysis with the question of what the eye is, over and above a collection of cells. A reflection upon the eye shows us that it is a circle in the face that opens up towards the world. I open my eyes and the world is there, I close them and it disappears as a visual display. The eye is also somehow connected to the idea of the person. When we meet the gaze of another, we feel that they are *there*, behind the eyes. There are many descriptions in literature and art of the eyes and the person being intimately connected. We have this notion, according to Sheets-Johnstone, because we have the bodily experience of closing our eyes and finding ourselves on the 'inside', behind our closed lids. When we close our eyes, we enter a realm of solitude, privacy and seclusion. Because we can retreat from the world and be with ourselves in this private way, we assume that others have access to the same kind of inner space. The experience of solitude, behind closed eyes, becomes transformed into an idea of interiority, which becomes more and more refined until we find the modern notions of subjectivity and personhood. The transformation from the bodily experience of eyes as circles shutting out the world to the sophisticated notion of subjectivity is an example of how body and bodily experiences play an important part in realms of meaning which have not traditionally been associated with the body.

On a cultural level, Sheets-Johnstone continues her analysis of the eye to show how the eye gives rise to notions of holiness. There are magic circles in a variety of religious rites, such as the pagan worship at Stonehenge, Buddhism and the rites of the Navajo Indians. One of the most striking examples of holiness connected to the eye can be found in the Buddhist ritual of the mandala, which has been practised for thousands of years. One type of mandala is a round pattern of sand in different colours and patterns, created by Buddhist monks during a long period of prayer and meditation. The end result, a meticulously patterned colourful work of art, is ceremoniously mixed together so that the colourful pattern becomes reduced to a grey mass, which is then simply swept away. In this way, the mandala illustrates the finite nature of things. Sheets-Johnstone draws attention to the way in which the mandala is described, as a circle meant to hold out that which is outside and keep together that which is within. The parallel to the eye is obvious.

The experience of vision thus allows us to develop notions of inwardness, solitude, subjectivity and holiness. We open our eyes and receive the world. Metaphors of light and clarity have often been used in connection with knowledge and understanding. The term *theoria* used by the ancient Greeks means literally seeing, where seeing and knowing (theory) are intimately connected. In many languages, we say 'I see' when we mean 'I understand'. The universal body experience of vision as light and clarity (as opposed to darkness and obscurity) is transformed and reproduced culturally in terms of abstract notions such as knowledge and understanding.

The linguist Mark Johnson (1987) focuses on the bodily, perceptual basis of language and reason. He argues against the objectivist theory of meaning in favour of a theory of meaning that is grounded in bodily experiences. These bodily experiences are organised in terms of what he calls 'image schemata', which are abstract patterns of experience and understanding that are preconceptual and prelinguistic. These patterns exist first as bodily experiences, but are gradually externalised and reproduced in a variety of linguistic and cultural expressions, resembling Sheets-Johnstone's examples. As soon as we attempt to communicate about image schemata we are forced to use language (prepositional speech). But this should not confuse us as to the nature of image schemata. They are *pre*linguistic, although we must use language to describe them. A person standing upright experiences being balanced on two feet. This experience is neither cognitive nor thematically reflected upon, but if we want to communicate about this experience we will use language. However, we must not mistake our way of describing things for the things described. The lived experience of standing upright on two feet is the bodily source of the externalisation we find in metaphors describing people as 'balanced' or, conversely, 'unbalanced'. We know what this metaphor means because we have the prelinguistic experience of standing upright.

In order to exemplify how understanding is grounded in bodily, prelinguistic experiences, Johnson (1987) analyses an interview with a man about rape. His analysis shows that the entire interview is structured around a metaphor which he calls 'physical attraction is a physical force' (p. 7). Without an implicit understanding of this metaphor it is not possible to *understand* what the man is saying. Every comment the man makes is comprehensible only if we have an understanding of the underlying metaphor that physical attraction is a physical force. We do not need to be thematically aware of the metaphor, but it underlies the structure of the text. For example, the man says: 'She's *giving off* very feminine, sexy *vibes* … I'm supposed to stand there and *take it* … The woman has *forced me* to turn off my feelings … they have *power over* me just by their presence …' (p. 7, italics in original). The underlying metaphorical structure is that the woman's appearance exerts a physical force which can cause things to happen in the world, in this case causing the man to do things that are outside his control. The logic of the narrative is thus that the woman is responsible for how she looks, and since physical attraction is a physical force, it is she and not the man who bears responsibility for the rape.

The point of the above example is to show that bodily experiences, patterned into metaphorical structures, underlie our understanding of linguistic, propositional statements. In order to understand the interview about rape, we must have a bodily experience about what the metaphor externalises. We know what 'force' is because our bodies exist in the material world. We have felt the wind blow hard against us, as small children we have been knocked over by brothers and sisters, we can feel force in our own bodies when our bladders are full or we need to vomit and so on. From these bodily experiences of force we build an understanding of force that not only refers to concrete experiences of mechanical force but also becomes metaphorised to include force on a psychological level. We speak of 'group pressure' and coercion. The initial bodily experience of force is the basis for a variety of meanings which we no longer associate with the body. We use bodily experiences in order to create categories of understanding that go beyond the realm of the body. We make use of the body *in order to understand*. This is far from the objectivistic theory of meaning. The body plays a crucial role in meaning and understanding.

The image schema of containment is based on one of our most fundamental bodily experiences, that of being a separate entity inside our skins. We are confined by boundaries which regulate inside and outside. Food enters the body through the mouth, passes through the body and exits as excrement. The experience of inside and outside of the body is the source of our understanding of containment. From this basic bodily experience we create the useful image schema of in–out. This schema is used when we have an understanding of something being contained in something else, when we set up boundaries, include and exclude and so on. From the in–out schema we develop the concept of transitivity: for example, if I am *in* my bed and my bed is *in* my bedroom, I understand that I am in the bedroom. The in–out schema fixes boundaries, and from this insight I can experience that things have a fixed place that is stationary. Because of this fixity in space, I gain the understanding of where things are *for me*. We move from a bodily sensation of containment to a metaphorised level of understanding that goes beyond the physical experience. We can often find the bodily basis of language if we become attuned to the way in which metaphors that guide our understanding are built upon prelinguistic bodily experiences (see Lakeoff & Johnson 1980).

Several authors within the phenomenological tradition besides Merleau-Ponty have pointed out the important role the body plays in understanding. Hans Jonas (1966) reflected on how different sensory modes (seeing, hearing, touching) are the bodily basis for many of our loftiest ideas that we do not initially associate with the body. For example, he calls sight 'the noble sense'. We have already seen how vision and light have been associated with understanding and knowledge. Jonas's analysis of sight gives us an insight into why this is so. He describes sight as the sense that gives us simultaneity of presence. I look at a landscape and the world is *there*, spread out before me. At once I have access to a view that is fixed and enduring through time. Sight is unique among the senses in this respect, since the other senses (hearing, taste, smell and touch) are all temporally dependent and non-spatial simultaneously. For example, in hearing, my auditory experience is dependent upon the duration of whatever produces the sound. I hear a dog barking, a car door slamming, someone whistling in the street outside my window. Hearing puts me in contact with an ongoing event over time. Hearing is dependent upon an outside event and the ability of consciousness to synthesise a series of impressions over time. Not only is hearing temporally determined, it is also a passive experience, in that the sound forces itself upon the hearer. I cannot choose not to hear in the same way that I can choose not to see, by closing my eyes or looking away. The event that produces sound is outside my control, which means that I am always open to sounds. I have no 'ear lids' that I can close and thus I must always be ready to hear, whether I wish to or not.

Touch is different from hearing, although it too is a temporally dependent sense. I cannot touch the entire object at once in the same way as I can see everything all at once. I must investigate the object sequentially with my hands in order to have a tactile experience. Objects stay put during the time I touch them (if they are not living things); they do not disappear suddenly in the way that a noise can suddenly stop when the

67

source ceases to produce the sound. To touch something demands activity on my part. I cannot be passive and have a tactile experience. I can be touched passively, but the sense of touch as a source of knowledge is an active one. My active encounter with the touched object gives the experience of the world as three-dimensional, since I move my body in relation to the object. But the sense of touch is still limited to a process over time, since I must investigate the object sequentially.

Through sight I gain an entirely different sense of the world's depth, and this experience is not limited in time. Only sight gives us the whole world at once, as long as we wish to experience it. I open my eyes and the world is there. Hearing is dependent upon events outside my control and touch demands an activity on my part during a specific temporal duration. Sight allows me to take in a scene in a neutral, non-engaged manner as long as I wish. I do not need to engage bodily with the seen objects, nor is what I see dependent upon something outside my control that can suddenly disappear. An object may move beyond my vision, but there is immediately something else to look at. This detached freedom of observation is the bodily basis of one of our dearest notions, according to Jonas, the idea of objectivity. I can observe without getting involved. The fact that I can take in an entire view that endures through time makes it possible to discriminate between what is continuous and what changes. Only the experience of sight gives us the possibility of maintaining a simultaneous presence and thus registering that which endures and that which changes. Due to this experience, we have the idea of a 'here' and 'there', a 'now' and 'then'.

Two further aspects of sight that Jonas emphasises are what he calls *dynamic neutralisation* and *distance*. Dynamic neutralisation has to do with the fact that neither the observer nor the observed is in any way changed by looking. Both hearing and touch involve a contact between the subject and the object of hearing or touch. Sound forces itself upon me; I cannot choose not to hear nor control the source of the sound, its genesis or its end. In touch, I force myself upon the object. I must bring my body into direct physical contact with the object in order to have a tactile experience. The unique indifference of sight gives me freedom, since I can be neutral and uninvolved in what I see, and in control of the scene through my ability to change views or shut my eyes. Sight is thus the freest and least dependent sense. Because of dynamic neutralisation we have the possibility of selective attention. I may observe any part of the view, when I wish, independently of activity from my side (touch) or temporally dependent events from the world (hearing).

The other important aspect of sight that gives it 'nobility' is distance. Distance is the form of presentation that objects afford in the experience of vision. Objects show themselves simultaneously and provide us with depth and distance. The visual field is presented as something my body can traverse. Our experiences of moving towards goals, or going 'forward' in a process, are based upon this fundamental experience of the body moving through a visual field. Finally, sight gives us the experience of a horizon, a continuation beyond that which we see before us. I experience a 'beyond' although it is not visually present. No one believes that the world ends at the border of what is seen in the present view from a determinate position. Even small children can understand that beyond their street lies another street, even if they cannot see it at the moment. There is always a 'beyond' presented in every visual horizon. There is no counterpart to this in hearing or touch. I can only replace my present hearing or touching with another hearing and touching which follows temporally. Jonas writes that the horizon we experience in sight is the bodily basis for a variety of noble ideas such as the eternal, the absolute and the idea of God. Jonas (1966) writes:

> Simultaneity of presentation furnishes the idea of enduring present, the contrast between change and the unchanging, between time and eternity. Dynamic neutralization furnishes form as distinct from matter, essence as distinct from existence, and the difference of theory and practice. Distance furnishes the idea of infinity. Thus the mind has gone where vision has pointed (p. 153).

We have seen that there are many reasons for re-evaluating the role of the body in meaning constitution and understanding. The body and knowledge are intimately related, despite our attempts to exclude the body from science and philosophy. The body is not the vessel of the soul, nor a deceiving trickster, but the living source of meaning and experience. If we regard the body in this way, it is obvious that this has implications for the relationship between body and self. I do not 'have' a body, I 'am' body and because of this, the body must be understood in a new way. Modern medicine has extensively investigated the container, machine-body, but the lived body has not yet been properly understood. I now turn to the issue of body and self.

3.2.2 The body and self

Because human beings are embodied, there is no 'view from nowhere'. The nature of human existence is to be situated within a perspective that has its origin in the body. It is from the body-as-centre that the world shows itself to us. Our access to the world is possible in and through perception, an achievement that involves an encounter between the embodied human being and the world. This encounter is reciprocal. The world is not only given to me, I am also 'given' in perception. Merleau-Ponty (1945/1962) writes:

> If I draw the object closer to me or turn it round in my fingers in order 'to see it better', this is because each attitude of my body is for me, immediately, the power of achieving a certain spectacle, and because each spectacle is what it is for me in a certain kinaesthetic situation. In other words, because my body is permanently stationed before things in order to perceive them and, conversely, appearances are always enveloped for me in a certain bodily attitude. In so far, therefore, as I know the relation of appearances to the kinaesthetic situation, this is not in virtue of any law or in terms of any formula, but to the extent that I have a body, and that through that body I am at grips with the world (p. 303).

The telephone is to my right and the window to my left. This 'being situated' is such a fundamental aspect of perception that it is hardly noticed. In order for the world to be perceived as ordered and myself as oriented, I must simultaneously perceive myself *in* situations. Thus the phenomenon of perception presupposes the insertion of my body into the scene. The implicit knowledge of 'where I am' (the so-called indexical 'here') is a tacit yet necessary term in the experience of perception. This implicit understanding of myself in the situation is at the deepest level the source of my experience of myself.

Merleau-Ponty calls the primordial embodied point of view underlying perception *le moi naturel* (the natural me). The natural self establishes our first contact with the world, before the complex edifice of the psychosocial self is built, although it is impossible to discern a strict boundary between the natural and the cultural self, as these levels are intertwined in humans. Merleau-Ponty (1945/1962) again:

> It is impossible to superimpose on man a lower layer of behaviour which one chooses to call 'natural', followed by a manufactured cultural or spiritual world. Everything is both manufactured and natural in man, as it were, in the sense that there is not a word, not a form of behaviour, which does not owe something to purely biological being – and which at the same time does not elude the simplicity of animal life ... through a sort of leakage and through a genius for ambiguity which might serve to define man (p. 189).

In our everyday usage of the term 'self' we most often refer to the psychosocial self, including self-consciousness, personality and character traits, memories, goals, values, affiliations to class, genus, ethnicity and so on. In the literature, the notion of self is highly ambiguous. Strawson (1999, p. 484) has discerned 21 different concepts of self. A variety of authors in different disciplines have various concepts of self, which makes the topic difficult and somewhat confusing (see Taylor 1989 and Zahavi 1999, 2005 for interesting reading on the self).

Zahavi (2005, pp. 101–110) summarises the different notions of self in terms of (1) the Kantian category (the self as a pure identity pole), (2) the hermeneutical perspective (the self as a narrative construction) and (3) the phenomenological perspective (the self as an experiential dimension). The Kantian notion of self has to do with the continuity of identity through time. One and the same subject gives coherence to the flow of diverse moments and renders these diverse moments as belonging to this one and the same subject. I am the same person who walked to school with a red lunch-box on my first day there, although there is very little that is similar between that 6-year-old girl and the self I experience today. The Kantian notion of self is an abstract notion, defining the subject as the pole towards which all experience past, present and future coincides. The hermeneutical perspective denies a self-given pole of identity and problematises this abstract, constant self in favour of the notion of the self as a construction, continually in the making. According to this view, the self evolves and changes according to our projects and our self-understanding. The self is thus a narrative construction, a story we tell ourselves about ourselves, lacking the solidity of the Kantian identity. It is highly sensitive to social interaction and can be understood as co-constituted by others to a large degree. Language, sociocultural norms and values have a significant bearing on how one defines oneself.

The phenomenological perspective takes its point of departure in the structure of experience. The self is the pole of experience that is implicitly given in perception. There is always a subject who is experiencing. In the experiencing there is an experiencing subject. The self is thus a permanent, necessary dimension of experience. The subject lives various experiences, experiences that have different qualities for that particular subject. They are lived and understood in the first person, as being interesting, boring, funny, sad, frightening and so on. There is someone who is experiencing X, and it is experienced in a certain way. The first-person perspective on one's own experiences is the core of the phenomenological understanding of the self. To be a self is to be an experiencing subject, and this form of existence is fundamentally grounded in the body and perception. Zahavi (2005) stresses that the self cannot be understood as something over and above experience, rather the self 'is present to itself precisely and indeed only when worldly engaged' (p. 126). He recommends replacing the notion of 'the subject of experience' with 'the subjectivity of experience' in order to emphasise the interconnectedness of self and world.

To be a person, or self, is to be a locus of experience that is unique. Our uniqueness has to do with our embodiment. There is no one else who is me, who can ever be me or replace me, as I am uniquely this embodied person at this particular point in time in this particular situation. Levinas (1969, 1987) founds his ethics on a similar insight, exemplified in the profound experience of looking into the face of the other. In the other's face I experience the transcendence of the other. He is beyond me, distant as another world. The other cannot be reduced to anything in my own experience, he is beyond any idea I can have of him. In his absolute otherness, the other constitutes a call, according to Levinas, an imperative not to kill, not to manipulate, not to oppress. The otherness of the other person, discovered in the epiphany of the face, is the ground of ethical behaviour. The fact that we are embodied selves, unique in space and time, constitutes the dignity of the human being. If we were not this unique point of view, incarnated in flesh, there would be no ground for the universal human dignity (*Menschenwürde*). As long as we exist, we are worthy of respect, even when other sources of dignity can no longer be applied (see Nordenfelt, this volume, Chapter 2).

The human self that is universal and worthy of respect is the incarnated point of view, the embodiment that opens up upon a unique field, a realm that goes by the name of 'subjectivity' in various philosophical and psychological traditions. From a Merleau-Pontian perspective, subjectivity is not tied to a specific state of mind or certain cognitive capacities, but rather understood as the source and upsurge of existence. Without subjectivity, no human experience and no human world. Subjectivity is a permanent field that exists as long as the human body exists. The body is always intrinsically connected to the human world, even if this lived body has lost some of the dimensions that we associate with the psychosocial self. Thus, even when the 'dignity of identity' (Nordenfelt, this volume, Chapter 2) is threatened by illness, injury and old age, we still have what could be called the 'dignity of subjectivity'. As long as I live, I am an incarnated subject, worthy of respect as an embodied human being, a unique point of view in the world. Merleau-Ponty (1945/1962) writes:

> In so far as, when I reflect on the essence of subjectivity, I find it bound up with that of the body and that of the world, this is because my existence as subjectivity is merely one with my existence as a body and with the existence of the world, and because the subject that I am, when taken concretely, is inseparable from this body and this world (p. 408).

The dignity of subjectivity is the dignity implicit in the embodied, first-person point of view. According to phenomenological thinking, this level of dignity must be regarded as primordial, that is to say, prior to any conceptualisations of dignity that are based upon psychological traits or social achievements. The dignity of subjectivity has to do with the uniqueness of the lived body, and in a sense is another way of describing the universal human dignity. The notion of dignity that has its source in subjectivity is based upon the recognition that every human being represents a unique, subjective point of view, a view that is incarnated in the lived body. A dead person cannot enjoy the dignity of subjectivity, since the unique, first-person perspective vanishes the instant the body dies (see Chapter 8). However, is the dignity of subjectivity something that all living human beings enjoy, or are there limits to and degrees of this form of dignity? This depends upon how one defines subjectivity and the first-person perspective.

Following Merleau-Ponty, I would argue that the subjectivity of the human being is not limited to cases where there is self-consciousness or a specific degree of conscious awareness. A sleeping person is still a subject. A person in a coma is still a subject. Even in sleep and in a coma, the lived body is still 'constituting meaning', although this level of meaning is not the meaning we traditionally refer to when we use the word. The dreamer dreams and the comatose person has experiences: people who have awakened from a coma can relate that they were experiencing during the coma. We speak of 'awakening' from a coma, which points towards its similarities with sleep. In fact, it is common practice in intensive care units that health-care professionals never discuss comatose patients in their presence, since it is possible that they may be aware of what is said. So even in altered states of consciousness, we still find the subjectivity of the lived body, and this subjectivity is not tied to the fact that the sleeper wakes up or the comatose patient comes out of the coma, but rather has to do with the fact that there is a *locus of experiencing*, however far from our normal experiences this experience may be. But is there really no limit to subjectivity? What about the brain-dead person? This is a difficult question. Because the lived body is not to be understood as a vessel containing consciousness, I would be inclined to argue that even the brain-dead person is a 'lived body' since the body continues to experience, in some way, although now on an extremely low level. Can we find a 'first-person perspective' in the brain-dead patient? There is no electrical activity in the brain, yet the heart is still pumping. Do we want to maintain that the person has died but the body lives? This dualistic way of expressing oneself goes entirely against the concept of the lived body argued for in this chapter. The debate about brain-death vs death defined as irreversible circulatory–respiratory failure illustrates the philosophical and ethical difficulties involved in a definition of death that proclaims a person to be 'dead' who in fact is still alive, in a purely biological sense. We do not need to pursue this difficult limit case here; suffice it to say that the notion of the dignity of subjectivity pertains to almost all cases of human embodiment in various stages of 'consciousness'.

The question as to whether animals have 'dignity' can be discerned in the debate about their ability to feel pain or not. We intuitively want to apply ethical standards to our behaviour towards animals that can feel pain in relation to slaughter, for example. We do not have the same concern when we poison a wasps' nest or kill ants. This concern we have about animals that can feel pain can be comparable to a wide notion of dignity (as living creatures), but animals do not possess the dignity of subjectivity since their self-consciousness does not reach the human level. The least mentally developed human being is a subject, because of their human nature, while the most highly developed animal is not a subject, at least not in the way subjectivity is understood in this context. That animals may have a rudimentary 'point of view' is conceivable, but this point of view is in principle out of our reach, as we cannot cross over into animal consciousness. So for the purposes of this book, the notion of subjectivity is reserved for human beings.

3.2.3   The lived body of older people

Simone de Beauvoir (1972) wrote: 'The vast majority of mankind looks upon the coming of old age with sorrow or rebellion. It fills them with more aversion than death itself' (p. 77). Her detailed account of the degeneration of the ageing body has now, some 30 years later, become a standard horror vision of old age in Western society. The wide-spread practice of plastic surgery for non-medical (cosmetic) purposes, increased interest in health foods and health spas, the pervasive commercial recommendations to lose weight and get into shape, all point towards the modern cultural preference for youth, health and beauty. In this cultural environment, ageing, and specifically the ageing body, is seen as something foreign, something to be resisted. Since we do in fact achieve better health and live longer than previous generations, this project does not seem as impossible as it might have seemed for someone living only 100 years ago. However, despite the increased chances of a healthy old age, no one can avoid the ageing process. Youthful beauty vanishes. The body becomes weaker, sicker and less dependable. Our mental capacities diminish. In old age we may even experience dementia, which, in its advanced stages, robs us of our personal self, understood in terms of a coherent narrative of memories, sense of self over time, values and so on. Besides the bodily and psychical changes involved in ageing, older people can experience the social stigmatisation of old age. The term 'ageism' refers to negative attitudes attributed to older people, simply because they are older. Older people can feel worthless, uninteresting, useless, a burden to others. Segregation, isolation and self-contempt can rob people of the very will to live. So, on a physical, mental and social level, old age is a challenging time.

The lived body of the ageing person cannot be understood simply by examining the brute corporeality of the objective body; rather, one must investigate how this particular aged body is lived. How does the person experience the physical, psychological and social changes and challenges of old age? Medical and sociological research on old age has tended to neglect the lived experience of older people, viewing the ageing body as either an objective machine-body or a field of play for socially constructed power discourses. Phenomenological studies (RimShin et al. 2003; Fleming & Russell 2004; Higgins 2005; Bullington 2006; Russell 2007) aim at elucidating the experience of ageing and thereby enabling us to learn more about what it is like to be an older person.

The lived body of the ageing person can be described as a changed life-world where previous capacities and roles are called into question. In my study (Bullington 2006) I found that older people reacted to the changes in their bodies and social situation in ways that did not correspond to objective descriptions of bodily dysfunction. One group of respondents experienced frustration in relation to the limitations of ageing and experienced their bodies as 'not me'. The body stood in the way of the will, which gave rise to the need for coping strategies. The aches and pains described in this group were in no way more severe than those described by the other respondents in the study, but these people experienced their disabilities as a battle between body and self. Hands that 'won't do what I want any more' (p. 164) and 'My body doesn't do what I want it to

73

do' (p. 164) illustrate how the body has become an alien thing, rather than one with the self. Another group of respondents, with similar health problems, had a different way of living their bodies, where health problems were accepted in a philosophical way: 'I have the insight that I am getting old, and I accept that. I know that I will have less and less energy and all of that, but I see it as a part of a natural process' (p. 164). The study showed that the mere fact of having aches and pains, altered appearance and changed social roles did not in itself necessarily lead to suffering. The way in which these changes were lived constituted the difference in how the aged body and self were perceived (see Bullington 2006 for further results and conclusions drawn from this study).

If we subscribe to the phenomenological perspective on the self as incarnated subjectivity, until the very last moment of life, we find that human beings have the dignity of subjectivity even when they are ill, disoriented and lacking in what can be characterised as a 'personal self'. This means that neither competence, health, wisdom nor merit plays a part in defining the dignity of human beings as embodied subjects. I have thus further articulated human dignity in terms of incarnated subjectivity. Let us now examine what this perspective means in terms of health care.

3.3   *Implications for health care*

It is known that the more patients lose their 'personality' the easier it is for them to be treated as just a case or a body part ('Can you check up on the hip in 5C?'). It is in general considered lower status in Western culture to work in geriatrics or psychiatry, areas of health-care specialisation that have in common the deterioration of the patient's psychosocial self. If being ill is a traumatic experience, then being ill in ways that break down one's 'merit' is even more traumatic. What does the dignity of subjectivity understood in terms of the lived body bring to this issue to help us to understand that the human being is infinitely precious and unique, simply by being an embodied human being?

The care and treatment of those who no longer possess the dignity of merit require an alternative way of conceptualising subjectivity and personhood in order to preserve an ethical standard in the relationship between patients and health-care professionals. When we no longer find the personality of the patient intact, it is easy to fall into an objectification of the person, a depersonalisation that can, at worst, lead to neglect, contempt and even violence. It has been suggested in this chapter that we need to modify our concepts of subject and subjectivity in order to include the notion of the subject as a *source of experience*, regardless of how bizarre or disintegrated that experience may seem in our eyes. The embodied subject is always a unique point of view, simply by being a lived body, and as such worthy of dignity and respect. Even if a confused older man cannot recognise his wife or follow the news, he has experiences of his world. We do not need to understand his world or approve of it, but because he is an incarnated subjectivity, we must respect his experiences as a possible human world. How does this respect show itself? When we can no longer communicate at the level of personality, thoughts and memories, we can simply be there and care for this person, who is experiencing the world in a very different way from us.

Caring for people with diminished faculties and forms of disease and handicap that break down their personality places high demands on care staff. We can no longer rely on our usual ways of making contact, conversing and consoling. In these cases, we are challenged to be present to the afflicted person in a special way. It is beyond the scope of this chapter to go into this issue, but see other chapters in this volume for some empirical examples of caring in such special circumstances.

References

Brentano, F. (1982) *Descriptive Psychology*. Felix Meiner Verlag, Hamburg.

Bullington, J. (2006) Body and self: a phenomenological study on the ageing body and identity. *Medical Humanities*, **32**, 25–31.

de Beauvoir, S. (1972) *The Coming of Age*. C.P. Putnam's Sons, New York.

Fleming, A.A. & Russell, C. (2004) 'Working it out': Older men remaking the lifeworld after stroke. *Royal Rehabilitation Centre Monograph Series* No. 8. University of Western Sydney, Sydney, Australia.

Higgins, I. (2005) The experience of chronic pain in elderly nursing home residents. *Journal of Research in Nursing*, **10**, 369–382.

Husserl, E. (1913/1962) *Ideas: General Introduction to Pure Phenomenology*, Vol. 1. Collier Books, New York.

Husserl, E. (1954/1970) *Crisis of European Sciences and Transcendental Phenomenology*. Northwestern University Press, Evanston, IL.

Johnson, M. (1987) *The Body in the Mind: The Bodily Basis of Meaning, Imagination, and Reason*. University of Chicago Press, Chicago.

Jonas, H. (1966) *The Phenomenon of Life, towards a Philosophical Biology*. Harper & Row Publishers, New York.

Lakeoff, G. & Johnson, M. (1980) *Metaphors We Live By*. University of Chicago Press, Chicago.

Levinas, E. (1969) *Totality and Infinity*. Duquesne University Press, Pittsburgh, PA.

Levinas, E. (1987) *Time and the Other*. Duquesne University Press, Pittsburgh, PA.

Merleau-Ponty, M. (1942/1963) *The Structure of Behavior*. Beacon Press, Boston, MA.

Merleau-Ponty, M. (1945/1962) *Phenomenology of Perception*. Routledge & Kegan Paul, London.

Merleau-Ponty, M. (1948/1964) *Sense and Non-Sense*. Northwestern University Press, Evanston, IL.

Merleau-Ponty, M. (1960/1964) *Signs*. Northwestern University Press, Evanston, IL.

Merleau-Ponty, M. (1964/1973) *Consciousness and the Acquisition of Language*. Northwestern University Press, Evanston, IL.

Merleau-Ponty, M. (1969/1973) *The Prose of the World*. Northwestern University Press, Evanston, IL.

Nagel, T. (1989) *View from Nowhere*. Oxford University Press, New York.

Plato (1961) *The Collected Dialogues of Plato* (eds E. Hamilton and H. Cairns). Princeton University Press, Princeton, NJ.

RimShin, K., YoungKim, M. & HyeKim, Y. (2003) Study on the lived experience of aging. *Nurse and Health Sciences*, **5**, 245–252.

Russell, C. (2007) What do older women and men want? *Current Sociology*, **55**, 173–192.

Sheets-Johnstone, M. (1990) *The Roots of Thinking*. Temple University Press, Philadelphia, PA.

Sheets-Johnstone, M. (1994) The body as cultural object/the body as pan-cultural universal. In: *Phenomenology of the Cultural Disciplines* (eds M. Daniel and L. Embree), pp. 85–113. Kluwer, Dordrecht.

Spiegelberg, H. (1982) *The Phenomenological Movement*. Martinus Nijhoff, The Hague.

Strawson, G. (1999) The Self and the SESMET. In: *Models of the Self* (eds S. Gallagher & J. Shear), pp. 483–518. Imprint Academic, Thorverton.

Taylor, C. (1989) *Sources of the Self*. MIT Press, Cambridge, MA.

Toombs, K. (ed.) (2001) *Handbook of Phenomenology and Medicine*. Kluwer, Dordrecht.

Zahavi, D. (1999) *Self-Awareness and Alterity*. Northwestern University Press, Evanston, IL.

Zahavi, D. (2005) *Subjectivity and Selfhood*. MIT Press, Cambridge, MA.

Part II   *Dignity and Older People: Some Empirical Findings*

4. *Dignity and Dementia: An Analysis of Dignity of Identity and Dignity Work in a Small Residential Home*

Magnus Öhlander

Introduction

This chapter is about dignity in the care of older people with dementia. Several kinds of dignity are elucidated by Lennart Nordenfelt in Chapter 2 of this book. One of these is human dignity (*Menschenwürde*). We all possess this kind of dignity from the fact that we as human beings are considered equals. As equals we have the same rights and obligations and should be treated in the same manner. Human dignity is fundamental and necessary in all kinds of care, and will therefore be touched upon in this chapter. However, the main focus is on what Nordenfelt designates dignity of identity. Like human dignity, dignity of identity exists even if the individual is not aware of it. A typical example of this, states Nordenfelt, is provided by the case of people with dementia. Dementia is a loss of several mental and everyday capacities, such as orientation in time and space, moral judgement, personal care and the ability to dress, and communication. This is caused by any of a number of diseases, among which Alzheimer's is one of the most common. 'These individuals are not aware of what happens around them. Nevertheless, we would say that their dignity could be violated' (Nordenfelt, this volume, Chapter 2).

In Nordenfelt's words, dignity of identity 'is the dignity we attach to ourselves as integrated and autonomous people, with a history and with a future, and with all our relationships to other human beings'. It is essential to dignity of identity that a person has an image of themselves as an individual with a past and a future and as a human being. Dignity of identity is connected to the person's physical self as well as lifestyle and culturally formed understanding of themselves.

The notion of 'dignity of identity' is not clearly separate from the comprehensive concept of identity widely used in cultural and social studies. A simple definition of identity is that it is the sum of the answers to questions such as 'How would I describe myself?', 'Among whom do I belong?', 'Where do I belong?' and 'What is my life story?' Identity is formed in the interplay between the individual, their social surroundings and the cultural and societal context in which they reside. Therefore the answer to the question of how someone would describe themself is dependent on the answers to questions such as 'How am I described by others?' and 'How does this person react to my actions?' In short, identity is an autobiographically informed characteristic of the self, positioned socially and inscribed in time and space (cf. Hellström, this volume, Chapter 5 and Lantz, this volume, Chapter 8). This definition of identity partly overlaps with the notion of dignity of identity. Furthermore, it is impossible to give a definition of identity or of the dignity of identity without including certain central cultural values. The dignity of identity is dependent on the upholding of values that together constitute what it is to be a human being. Which cultural values are to be included in a definition of identity or the dignity of identity probably varies depending on historical context, ethnicity, class and perhaps also sex and age.

Identity is an ongoing process. It can be reformed, weakened and violated. It continuously needs to be performed, communicated, elaborated, negotiated and symbolically shaped in several ways (e.g. Goffman 1990). This job of creating, recreating and upholding is summarised in the term 'identity work'. Identity work is accomplished in many ways. In fact, the ways in which a person dresses, walks, talks and eats communicate identity (as well as dignity) to the person themself and to others. Whether the person drinks coffee or not, has milk or sugar with it or not, likes biscuits or a pastry with it, or refers to a need to cut down on fat and sugar, says something about this person. The stories someone likes to tell to others, about themself or about someone else, say something about who this person is. If different people react to the same event with different feelings it may communicate something about each one of them. Every act, however small and insignificant it might be, is at the same time an act of communicating, elaborating and negotiating identity. If one accepts this description of what identity is, it means that the business of everyday life is crucial in identity work.

When identity work is performed in a decent way it upholds dignity and could be defined as 'dignity work'. Örulv & Nikku (2007) have described dignity work in dementia care as 'respecting, protecting, and maintaining the dignity of the residents'. They point out that 'what dignity work in dementia care consists of is by no means unequivocal, but involves a delicate act of balancing potentially conflicting values' (p. 510).

In this chapter I will focus on a particular form of dignity work: dignity of identity work. I have taken into account the fact that identity work is performed in the interaction between the individual subject and their physical, social and cultural environment. Of course this also goes for dignity of identity work. In a residential home for older people dignity of identity work is performed by the residents themselves, in their everyday interaction with each other and with the staff. Further, as will be shown, the physical environment and the routines of care interact with the residents' dignity work. The care of people suffering from dementia differs from 'ordinary' care in such a way that care in the residential home could be described as having been designed to reconstruct and maintain the abilities the residents have lost as a consequence of their dementia. In the residential home, then, it is most evident that dignity of identity work is performed by the staff on behalf of the residents. In this chapter I describe and analyse dignity of identity work as performed by the residents themselves, by the staff on behalf of the older people, and as interaction between individuals, their physical environment and the characteristics of everyday life.

Above, I attempted to show (1) that the dignity of identity is dependent on the maintenance of several culture-specific values; and (2) that these values are expressed and reproduced in the actions of everyday life (dignity of identity work). The primary aim of this chapter is to use ethnographic descriptions of dementia care in a residential home to outline which values or ideals constitute dignity, and how these values are staged, reproduced and managed in the everyday life of care. In other words, this chapter is about dignity of identity work. How is dignity 'made' in the daily life of the residential home?

In the care of people with dementia, the emphasis is placed on normality, the possibility of living a life that is as normal as possible. The secondary aim of this chapter is to discuss the connections between the hegemonic idea of normality and dignity of identity. What is the interplay between dignity and normality? Are they dependent on each other? Is dignity central to the understanding of normality, and vice versa?

Empirically, this chapter is based on a seven-month period of ethnographic fieldwork where participant observation was carried out in a small residential home to which I have given the fictitious name Danneholm. The observations were supplemented with interviews performed with the staff. Participant observation means that I was present in the residential home, taking notes while sharing and participating in the everyday life of the residents and staff. The fieldwork was organised to cover different periods of the year, hours of the day and situations and events in everyday life. My presence meant that I was involved in what happened at the residential home. Since I was a part of this everyday life, I let myself appear in the field notes as a self-evident and natural part of the daily social interaction in the residential home. By doing so I was able to account for and evaluate the effect of my presence. This means that I appear as one of several actors in the empirical illustrations given in this article. This is a common method in the field of cultural analysis. (For further information on this particular field work, see Öhlander 1999; for more about field work, participant observation and the role of the researcher, see e.g. Schatzman & Strauss 1973; Agar 1996; Halstead 2001.)

4.1 Living together in a residential home

A residential home is a special type of care that could for instance be designed for people with dementia. The ideal residential home is small and homelike, with a small number of residents and round-the-clock staffing. The residential home described in this chapter, here called Danneholm, is in Stockholm, Sweden. It is located in an ordinary neighbourhood and consists of three merged flats in a building dating from the turn of the 20th century. At the time of the fieldwork six older women were living there, usually called 'the ladies' by the staff. Each of them had a room of her own. They shared three bathrooms, a smaller and a larger kitchen, a dining room, a drawing room and a living room. Their rooms were furnished with their own furniture, except for the beds, which were of the type found in hospitals. The common space was mostly furnished with furniture of an older style, from the first half of the 20th century. All in all the rooms were decorated in a way that was intended to be pleasant, comfortable and homelike. As well as the private rooms and the communal spaces there was one smoking room and one office, both mainly intended for the staff.

Within these walls the six ladies spent most of their time. They mostly had the daily company of each other and the staff. Sometimes a relative visited, but not very often. The ladies did not know each other before they all moved to the residential home. Now they lived together, slept and woke up under the same roof, ate most meals together, watched TV, took care of the activities of everyday life inside a shared home. They all had some kind of neurological or psychological condition. Sometimes they seemed to enjoy each other's company, sometimes they did not. In one way or another they made a clear distinction between themselves, the residents, on the one hand, and the staff on the other. They seemed to prefer the company of the staff.

Being together was an important ideal in the residential home. At all hours of the day and on every occasion the staff tried to make the residents be together and enjoy each other's company. With regard to dignity of identity, this act of bringing the ladies into social interaction calls attention to the individual as a person with relationships to others. The basic idea is that all humans are better off in the company of others. Social interaction is of course also a condition that generates possibilities of expressing identity.

However, these ladies who had been brought together in this residential home had no common history. Except for the fact that they had lived through the same overall historical events (the depression of the 1920s, the Second World War, and so on), they had no or only limited mutual experiences before moving into the residential home. Once they were in the residential home their ability to share experiences and get to know each other was reduced because of their dementia. The ladies tried to classify themselves, the other residents and the staff. This outline of a kind of social map for the dwelling was never really finalised. One could characterise the old people's attempts as temporal. One example of this outlining of a social classificatory map was when Beata used the word *syster* in addressing a member of the staff. Like its English counterpart, the Swedish word *syster* has two possible meanings, sister and nurse. Probably she meant 'nurse' since on several occasions she spoke of a member of the staff as *syster* and she was a stickler for etiquette. The other residents mostly considered Beata as nice and pleasant. Fanny, on the other hand, was usually considered as troublesome or tiresome by the other ladies.

The ideal of being together was also threatened by the fact that not all of the residents really got along with each other. Now and then the ladies got into conflicts. They quarrelled and sometimes even came to blows. On several occasions Ylva and Christina got into a kind of slow and low-voiced quarrel. Mostly they seemed to be competing for the staff's favour, or perhaps Christina just tried to get the staff's attention to tease Ylva, who was very dependent on the staff. Christina, who had trouble speaking, could take hold of Ylva's arm and squeeze hard when she became angry. Ylva, in turn, repeatedly stated that Christina was an 'awful person'. Fanny's straightforward manner, sometimes even coarse language and vulgarity, often provoked the other residents. Often the staff put Fanny in another room, just to make sure there would not be any trouble. For instance, from time to time she had to eat her meals by herself in the kitchen, or watch TV on her own while all the others watched TV in another room.

One morning, when a church service was on TV, staff placed two armchairs close together right in front of the TV set. Anna and Emmy sat there enjoying the morning service. A few yards away sat Fanny on a green sofa. Christina came into the room and sat on a chair, close to Fanny. They were all listening to a woman singing. Christina kept time with her foot and seemed to be caught up in the music. Sometimes Fanny was also quiet, and when she spoke it was in a low voice. When the solo singing ended the priest took over and began to speak. The volume of Fanny's speech increased. Then the congregation joined in a hymn. Fanny tried to sing along. When the music stopped, Christina rapidly got up and walked out of the room. Before the priest had begun his sermon, Fanny started to talk. Even though she spoke really loudly, I could only hear fragments.

'You may stay here ... That one shut up ...'

Soon Fanny had competition from the priest. He was preaching and Fanny spoke loudly to herself.

One of the staff was in the nearby kitchen. She could hear Fanny.

'Now she's starting to create a disturbance in there', the nursing assistant said.

Anna turned her attention from the television to Fanny.

'Be quiet in church!'
'That one's an intolerable person', Emmy added.

Anna and Emmy started to discuss Fanny. I could only catch a few phrases.

'We don't like that one', Anna established.

The nursing assistant moved Fanny to the kitchen and nodded towards Anna and Emmy.

'Look how well they're getting on together.'

And they were. Now they were more occupied with talking about Fanny than with listening to the priest.

'The girls are doing well', one of them said.

Quite often Fanny created a stir. One morning she woke up at quarter to eleven. Two of the staff found her as she was walking down the corridor and took her to the bathroom. They let her go to the toilet and tried to help her into the shower. Fanny had not had a shower for a very long time, but the staff could not persuade her this time either. Half an hour later I could hear Fanny and Anna quarrelling in the kitchen and went to see what was going on. Fanny was standing close to the kitchen table and Anna was sitting on the settee. No one else was there. As Anna caught sight of me she said:

'Now I've got this one here again.'

She pointed her finger at Fanny.

'But I suppose the doctor will come and have a look at her, then he'll see.'

Fanny sat down on a chair, starting to sing loudly and persistently beat time with her hand on the kitchen table. I felt sorry for Anna and took her with me to join the others in another part of the house.

If being together was a foundation stone in the constitution of the meaning of good care and the dignity of identity, an important part of dignity work was simply to make the ladies interact and take part in the activities of the residential home. But, as illustrated above, pleasant and enjoyable togetherness could all of a sudden turn into more or less offensive behaviour. Thus an equally important part of dignity work was to make sure that this togetherness did not crack and turn into annoyance and quarrelling. Social interaction needed social order. And surveillance and keeping order was a palpable part of dignity work. In short, dignity work in the residential home was about regulating activities.

4.2   The homelike nature of the residential home

Its homelike nature is a primary framework of the residential home. Following Erving Goffman (1986) and his thesis on how to understand situations and strips of ongoing reality, a framework could be described as a specific understanding of a specific place and what is going on there. The ladies were supposed to be encompassed within the homelike frame – that is, to interpret the residential home as their home, the people living there as friends and their lives as quite normal. The staff also used another framework, one saying that this is a place for old people suffering from dementia. And in this framework the residential home is also a workplace and a site for special care. The ladies were denied access to the possibility of framing the residential home as a place of professional care. Not once, during seven months of fieldwork, did I hear the staff telling one of the ladies she had a disease and was living in a care unit. Still, since the framework of the place as a home where normal life was threatened by the ladies' own interpretations and by their conflicts, an ongoing out-of-frame activity (Goffman 1986) was necessary. Dignity work then took place as in-frame activities, in interaction with the residents, and in out-of-frame activities, concealed from the ladies. Mainly this out-of-frame activity was composed, as mentioned above, of surveillance and regulating activities. One example of this is to be found in the above discussion on keeping social order, demonstrated by the way in which the staff moved Fanny when she nearly ruined the atmosphere of homelike relations, togetherness and harmony.

Now and then the staff also had to cope with 'wrong' interpretations or bewilderment about what kind of place the residential home is. In the terminology of Goffman (1986), the ladies temporarily transformed the schema of interpretation called 'a home'. They kept the basic home-frame, but transformed it slightly. An illustration of this is the following. At a Swedish festival called 'Lucia' a group of children from a daycare centre

visited Danneholm. Dressed in white and carrying candles, the children sang the traditional Lucia songs. After this event I found Anna standing outside the door of her
room. She was just standing there, watching the closed door.

'What are you thinking about?' I asked her.

She pointed at her door.

'Well, that's my room. They're there now.'
'Who?' I wondered, but Anna didn't have the time to answer before I understood
whom she meant.
'Yes', I said, *'the children had a look at your room.'*
Anna looks at me.
'Who?'
'The children who sang those Lucia songs, they visited your room', I explained.
'Oh, did they sing? Well, I wasn't here then. I was at home.'
'You listened to the children singing.'
'Oh no. I was at home then. I was.'

She looked confused, so I agreed with her version.

Anna spoke about 'my room' as she stood in front of the door. Who she meant when she
said that someone was in her room, we will never know. After I started to talk about the
children Anna spoke about her 'home' as if it was somewhere else and not Danneholm. On
another day during my fieldwork Anna was sitting on a sofa when she suddenly stood up,
walked out into the corridor and said she had to milk the cows. She could have meant
something else, just didn't find the right words, or she could have temporarily been deci-
phering the everyday world as if she were somewhere else in time and space.

Another episode, illustrating an alternative interpretation of the place and what is
going on, occurred one afternoon when some of the ladies and staff were watching TV
in the living room. After a few moments Christina stood up and walked away. Beata's
door opened. The light was out in her room, it was all dark. For a while the door stood
open, no one was visible in the room. Suddenly Beata came out of the room. She looked
very serious. With the help of her wheeled walking frame, she walked away. She didn't
say anything. When she passed behind the group watching TV it looked as if she was
unaware of their presence. One of the staff smiled at Beata and said:

'Hello, Beata!'

Beata remained grave and didn't say anything.

'Is there anything you need?' the member of staff asked.

Beata answered briefly,

'No.'

She walked away. After a few minutes she returned, and walked behind the ladies
watching TV on her way back to her room. Loudly she said:

'No, it's wrong! Everything's wrong!'

and returned to her room. We went on watching TV. Beata came out of her room for a second walk around. This time I said hello to her and she returned my greeting. When she got to Ylva they shook hands and exchanged polite phrases. Beata completed her second round of the home and passed me on her way back. Her face was close to mine when she whispered:

'Look out! Look out, because it's all a fake, you see.'

I didn't know what to answer, just smiled and nodded.

Except for Beata herself, no one could really know what she meant. Perhaps the whole residential home was a fake. Or maybe she was in her own world and was talking about something only she knew. During the fieldwork some of the ladies repeatedly talked about Danneholm as their home and the next moment as if they were guests in someone else's home. At dinner Beata could thank everyone for visiting her and then express her gratitude for being invited. The here-and-now of the residential home could all of a sudden become a part of something else, for instance of a reality where Emmy had to hurry up and prepare dinner before her husband came home from work.

In everyday life everyone needs to interpret new surroundings and experiences in order to classify them, to know what to think about the whole and what to do. In a way the residential home seemed to be a more or less constant new experience for the ladies living there. Or perhaps it would be more accurate to say that they could never really entirely endorse the home-frame presented to them. To the ladies, one may assume, the homelike nature of the place at the same time represented a kind of cosy and pleasant safeness and a deceptive framework they could never trust as being real, or be sure was not another reality in another time and space.

In other words, the everyday reality of the residential home, the shared world of the ladies, was a fragile reality. It involved constant work of interpretation. The staff managed this fragile reality in different ways. While the ladies strove the whole time to make sense of themselves, of the other residents, of the staff and of the place where they all spent their days, the staff interpreted the interpretations and doings of the residents. This was one of the most important out-of-frame activities. The staff could correct 'wrong' interpretations, they could separate the residents when they didn't get along and threatened to crack the image of a pleasant time together at home, or they could just play along. This presupposed surveillance and checking of how reality was interpreted and what the ladies were saying and doing. All in all, this was how this fragile reality was kept on its feet. And keeping up the framework of the homelike nature of the place was an important ingredient in dignity work. It kept the context of care together. In this context, business as usual was possible.

Perhaps the home-frame could be seen as a benign fabrication, with the setting and the staff as the primary fabricators (Goffman 1986). Still, the staff talked about the residential home as a home, and I suppose they would all have said it really was a home. The home-frame was never intended as a fabrication, it was understood as the primary frame in which this place and its activities should be understood.

4.3 Activities and routines

As stated in the introduction, dignity of identity is not just something someone has or could obtain once and for all. It needs to be maintained. The appearance of being together and the sense of living at home as usual were parts of this maintenance work. So also was the well-embraced value of being active. Being active is a key value in the care of older people, as in society as a whole. According to this value, rather than being inactive it is better to do something, even just a hobby or occupation that does not really contribute to the well-being of society or anything else. The staff at Danneholm some-times complained about the residents being lazy, 'just sitting on their heavy bottoms'. The ideal of being active was realised in that the ladies took part in the business of everyday life. These activities were ordered into routines that were supposed to give sense to orientation in time.

The days in Danneholm followed a specific rhythm, a repeating order in which the ladies had to take part. In the morning the staff usually gathered in the small kitchen, discussed miscellaneous subjects, got reports from the night staff, exchanged and dis-cussed the latest experiences of the ladies and planned the day. The residents got up at different times; usually Christina and Anna were first. Fanny woke up long after the others. As soon as they got up the ladies sat down in the small kitchen and were given a cup of coffee. Chat and laughter filled the room. The rest of the residential home rested in drowsiness and silence. About half past eight the sounds and activities became more intense. Behind the closed doors of the three bathrooms one could hear running water and voices. Those who were not doing their morning toilet lay in bed or walked about. The staff made the beds, collected the dirty laundry and tidied up in the ladies' rooms. About half past nine, when everything was in order, they all had breakfast in the dining room. Some of the ladies usually helped the staff lay the table and after breakfast they helped clear the table and wash up. When one of the ladies set the dinner table, for instance, the staff made it as easy as possible, putting the cutlery, plates and glasses almost in order, just for the ladies to put everything in its right place. During dinner, one of the staff told me, one of the ladies might accidentally keep the butter knife, and put it in her mouth. The staff didn't say anything, just let her keep the knife. A nursing assistant said:

> *'They eat from the bowls of jam with the serving spoon. If they serve themselves some salad it sometimes happens that they keep the serving spoon and start eating with it. If this happens you just have to pretend that you haven't seen it, get a new spoon and put the old one aside. But if they find out what you're doing they could get angry, even if you try to do it [hide the spoon] as discreetly as possible. Well, they discover that they've done something wrong. But most of the time it goes well.'*

Once, when one of the ladies cleared the table, she put the ice cream, butter and bread in the wall-cupboard where the household utensils are kept. One of the staff said that the lady was very happy and proud since she had cleared the table all by herself. Everything was left in the cupboard until she left the room. Sometimes one of the ladies would do the washing up after dinner. Some of them had poor eyesight, and the staff usually washed everything again, just to be sure it was properly done.

During the day the staff and the residents spent their time doing things people normally do. By and large they enjoyed each other's company, chatted, read the paper or a book, listened to music or watched TV. The staff had some administrative work to do. A large part of the time was spent on doing chores: apart from preparing food there were things like doing the laundry and looking after clothes, shopping and other errands. Thursday was house-cleaning day. This was the only occupation the residents never participated in. Almost every day some of the residents went for a walk, and most Wednesdays some of them, with staff, went on quite a long excursion. Every afternoon at about three o'clock they all had coffee. It was not unusual for them to linger for a while at the coffee table and eventually move to the living room and start to watch the evening programmes on TV. After dinner, around eight o'clock, the staff started to help the ladies with personal care and getting ready for bed. The staff who worked evenings left at nine, and after that only one member of staff was left: the nursing assistant on the night shift. The ladies went to bed at different times. Yvette and Emmy usually stayed up until eleven or twelve. Generally, by midnight only the night nurse was still up.

Daily life in Danneholm went on at an even pace, the same every day and week after week. Everyday activities established a routine with few surprises. Each day had its fixed times for getting out of bed, attending to bodily needs, having breakfast and lunch, watching TV and getting together for dinner. Some of the ladies sometimes helped out with all the chores that have to be done in a well-run household and home. The rhythm of the passing weeks was marked by the weekends, when there was more special food, and the year was mapped out by the major festivals such as Christmas, Easter and the celebration of midsummer.

This order was deliberate: it was intended to compensate for the residents' disorientation. 'Habits are the best support', the staff stated on several occasions. In other words, order in time and space and the repetition of behaviour was a cornerstone in the delivery of care. In short, one could say that the support of routine was a highly cherished ideal. Still, another ideal was that everyone was allowed to do as she liked. No one should be forced to participate in such activities as preparing food or setting the table. And no one should be forced to take a shower. Yet this ideal of doing as one likes constantly conflicts with the need for routine, the importance of keeping the body fit and clean, and the ideal of being active. Being active was an ideal embraced at Danneholm, as elsewhere in the care sector. One source of disagreement among staff and residents was the ladies' occasional unwillingness to participate, to keep up the routines and to be active.

The ordering of time and space was accompanied by the maintenance of the body. Much effort was put into keeping the residents' bodies clean and dressed. This was done in privacy; showers, the morning visits to the bathroom, and dressing were always private. The ladies' nails had to be trimmed, their hair had to be cut and styled. The staff spent time on looking after the ladies' hair and making sure that their clothes looked good. Some of the ladies were very careful with their appearance. They wanted to wear their jewellery and sometimes make-up.

Another bodily need is to eat good, tasty and nourishing food. The staff tried to control the residents' eating habits. For instance, they tried to cut down on the their consumption of sugar, and to make them eat more vegetables and less bread during meals.

The marking of time and all activities of everyday life were central parts of the ongoing dignity of identity work. Activities and routines that kept to time, the home nice and clean, the ladies well dressed and nourished and everyone meaningfully occupied: this implied a view of the residents as fully functional human beings, living ordinary lives and doing things normal people usually do. To the extent that the ladies gave impressions of themselves, more or less deliberately telling others who they were, their impression management (Goffman 1990) could rely on a sense of normality. And to the extent that other people's reaction to the ladies' presentations of themselves were relevant to these women's dignity of identity, the social and physical environment communicated that nothing was out of the ordinary.

4.4   *Identity*

One afternoon, after coffee, we were all looking at some photographs. Some of the photos were from a trip the staff had been on. Others were from Anna's birthday. The photos showed Anna surrounded by coffee-drinking ladies. On the table, in front of Anna, someone had placed a Swedish flag. Other photos showed Anna sitting on a chair in the kitchen, wearing her dressing gown. She looked as if she had just woken up, and was smiling and hugging her 'dog' (a soft toy). One of the staff showed Anna some of the photos and asked her:

'Who is this?'

Anna looked at the photos, thinking.

'Yes, who could that be?' she asked.

The staff said that Anna should be able to recognise the woman in the photos.

'No, I don't know', Anna declared.
'It's you.'
'Indeed. Well, I suppose I'm cleaning up as usual', Anna declared.

Anna had dementia and perhaps it was no big deal that she could not recognise herself in a photo. But she was asked if she did, and she was supposed, somehow or other, to find it relevant and interesting to be able to identify herself. Anna did not seem surprised it was her, and her comment said something about her: she was cleaning. The staff sometimes spoke about Anna's former employment as a housekeeper. Cleaning up was something she had probably done every day of her working life.

Knowledge about the ladies and their former lives was considered highly significant in the residential home. Gathering as much knowledge as possible about the clients is also a technique recommended in textbooks on the care of people with dementia. The staff gathered as much information as possible about the Danneholm residents. They got information from institutions where the ladies had lived previously, and from relatives and friends. The staff also asked the residents about their life and life histories, even though what they said was not considered totally reliable. This kind of information was used in everyday care; for example, to fill in the ladies' own narratives about themselves. This could be understood as an act of reconstruction of the ladies' life histories and presentations of self to others: in short, their identities as shown to and perceived by others.

Another use of this biographical knowledge was that these life stories helped the staff to understand why one of the residents was behaving or reacting in a certain way. One example of this was Ylva's lack of independence and need to be around the staff. One explanation of this was that she had been married to a dominant man and that her only role in their relationship had been that of a beautiful hostess. Another example was the difficulty of getting Fanny into the shower. The staff discussed the possibility that she had been abused as a child. One staff told me that Fanny was not comfortable being nude in the shower, in front of the staff. While in the shower, she spoke to the staff as if she thought they were men.

Of course the staff did not know the whole story about each resident. Even the ladies' children could not possibly know everything relevant about their parents. This means that the reconstruction of identity was done using fragments of life stories, and possibly even with pieces that were not entirely correct. In this sense the reconstruction contained components of construction. In fact no identity is wholly true or accurate in any 'objective' way: identity is always a kind of ongoing construction (e.g. Goffman 1990). These ongoing constructions always use pieces of the life story provided by a selective memory. Identity is always formed in relation to the interests at hand and the circumstances in a specific phase of life, or a specific situation in everyday life. In the case of these older people with dementia living in a residential home, the staff played an essential role in the identity processes. The staff (re)constructed the identities on behalf of the people with dementia, on the basis of what they knew about the residents.

Part of the reason for doing this is that it is in the interests of the smooth running of the residential home itself. One immediate concern was to get a grip on the social interactions between the ladies, and between them and the staff, and to be aware of different possible scenarios in the everyday context of care. In the words of Schutz (1975), the staff need typologies and recipes to make their life world of care comprehensible and manageable. From my field notes, and from the interviews with the Danneholm staff, I could easily identify a kind of 'typecasting'. One resident was repeatedly described as the one always hanging round the staff and always in need of their attention and sometimes protection from the other residents. Another was regarded as the wise, thoughtful, solid and independent one. Sometimes she was called 'the Madame'. Yet another lady was recurrently depicted as nice and friendly, but a recluse who preferred to stay in her own room. A fourth lady was often described as noisy, rude and disorderly, and yet charismatic and independent. Sometimes she was spoken of as 'the General'. In this way these residents were arranged in a typology and thus given specific roles that suited the residential home's context of social interaction and care. Their possibilities of presenting themselves to others – and in that way displaying their identity – were probably circumscribed by this typology, which ruled the everyday life of the residential home.

Of course the presentation of self in everyday life is always done within a specific framework that determines the possibilities of such presentation. When someone has

90

dementia their possibilities of doing well in a self-presentation are likely to be limited, or at least seen as limited by others. At the same time it is likely that their relatives and/ or the staff are more inclined to correct, fill in and supplement the self-presentations made by people with dementia. And in the residential home, where these people spend most of their time, the context of social interaction and care influences the possibilities and ways of presenting the self to others.

The ongoing interpretation of what the ladies did and said, and the use of reconstructions of their preferences, lives and experiences, was yet another ingredient in dignity work done by the staff. As dignity work this was a kind of surveillance and regularisation of activity to improve the residents' daily well-being and make the everyday life of the residential home run as smoothly as possible. Reconstructing the identities of people who supposedly cannot manage to maintain them on their own could also be seen as dignity work in another sense. Even though the reconstruction of someone else's identity necessarily partly includes innovations and novelties, the staff contributed to the ladies' possibilities of maintaining a sense-making identity.

4.5   Home, sweet home

As already mentioned, its homelike character was a central feature of Danneholm. Why was this so important? For one reason, the residential home was a part of a major shift from institutional care to in-home care. Even though the idea of the home as the best place for care is much older, in Sweden as elsewhere this trend has been going on since the 1950s, in the care of older people as well as in the care of people with mental health problems or disabilities. In Sweden, as in many other countries, 'the home' is a key symbol (cf. Ehn & Löfgren 2001; Löfgren 2003). A 'symbol' is described by Sherry Ortner (1973) as 'a vehicle for cultural meaning' (p. 1339). A symbol is a *key* symbol in that it is emphasised as important by the people under study; it frequently recurs in different contexts; no one is really indifferent to it; it is an object of cultural elaborations and/or it is surrounded with restrictions, clear guidelines and rules.

Ortner differentiates between two types of key symbols: *summarising symbols* and *elaborating symbols*. And there are two forms of elaborating symbols: *root metaphors* and *key scenarios*. Summarising and elaborating symbols are, Ortner proposes, two ideal types constituting ends of a continuum. 'The home', I would suggest, is both a summarising symbol and the kind of elaborating symbol conceptualised as a key scenario. Depending on situation and context, 'the home' functions as both kinds of symbol in the setting up of the residential home as a place of good care and as a place for dignity and dignity work.

Summarising symbols 'are those symbols which are seen as summing up, expressing, representing for the participants in an emotionally powerful and relatively undifferentiated way, what the system means to them' (Ortner 1973, p. 1339). This category of symbols 'includes all those items which are objects of reverence and/or catalysts of emotion' (p. 1340). 'The home' summarises central values, ideals and feelings such as privacy, autonomy, loving care, family, friends, being together, leisure, independence, security, relaxation, cosiness, creativeness, the 'I' and the presentation of self. As a symbol 'home' of course also contains more problematic aspects of life, such as gender inequalities, loneliness, isolation, injustice, difficult childhood memories, violence and assault. In the context of care it is mostly the more bright, pleasant, positive and salutary aspects that are emphasised. What makes 'the home' a *summarising* symbol is not only the fact that it sums up several, and to some extent contradictory, values, ideals and feelings but also the circumstance that it awakens a whole complex of feelings that are never actually elaborated, or do not need to be in every situation. Furthermore, as a summarising symbol 'the home' could be given different meanings by different individuals but still be a uniting symbol.

Seen as a summarising symbol, the traditional institution was usually described as a place where individuals became passive patients deprived of autonomy and personal identity. In contrast, 'the home' represents autonomy, the expression of the self and self-chosen activity (e.g. Öhlander 1999; Löfgren 2003; Öhlander 2007). If the traditional institution represents passivity, the home symbolises being able, having the possibility of conducting one's own life. Autonomy and self-chosen identity, based on life history, partly constitute dignity of identity. Perhaps being active on one's own terms is also related to dignity.

At the same time as 'the home' is used as a summarising symbol, it is also the type of elaborating symbol Ortner designates as a 'key scenario'. Elaborating symbols are those sorting out and organising complex experiences, ideas and values, 'making them comprehensible to oneself, communicable to others, and translatable into orderly action' (Ortner 1973, p. 1340). As mentioned, Ortner differentiates between two types of elaborating symbols. The root metaphor is a symbol that sorts out experience and provides a guidelines for the connections between different experiences and between experiences and culture. A key scenario has to do with what are desirable goals and how to think and act to achieve them. As a summarising symbol 'the home' has various and equivocal meanings and is emotionally charged. It is important, ambiguous, loaded with feelings and yet rather indistinct. As a key scenario 'the home' is advising, normative and requesting. In other words, as a key scenario 'the home' suggests how everyday life should be staged and lived, and how one should act to make this happen. For instance, activity, social intercourse and pleasantness, and an individual identity are central values and desirable goals. In this type of care, orientation in time and space can be added. The home as such, its design, equipment, furnishing and decoration, are some of the means used to reach these goals, to stage and reproduce these values over and over again.

Considering dignity of identity work, 'being homelike' should be understood not only as referring to a physical environment, or as a place, stage or scene for interaction, but also as a complex of guiding and sometimes compelling values. These values are clear and distinct and yet ambiguous and contradictory. As a symbol 'being homelike' is clear-cut and instantly recognisable and still indistinct and overcrowded with equivocal meaning. This is, I would suggest, what makes 'being homelike' culturally fundamental and attractive as an ideal in care. It makes dignity of identity possible, and at the same time an obligation. For example, it provides potential for the subject to exercise autonomy and possess an individually shaped sense of the 'I'. But the autonomic 'I' is also an obligation. This means that, compared to what might happen in a traditional institution, dignity of identity can suffer greater damage in a homelike context. Dignity work is easier in a homelike institution, and there should be a lesser risk of violating someone's dignity of identity. But if this does happen the effect could be more serious and deeply sensed. This implies that care is a more precarious task in a context characterised by its homelike nature.

4.6   Dignity, normality and culture

The kinds of dignity work described in this chapter uphold some of the characteristics of what it is to be human. Another way of looking at this dignity work is to say that it fends off the decline that could deprive someone of dignity of identity. In the description of dementia, a salient feature is often loss of ability. People with dementia lose their ability to orient themselves in time and space. They cannot always express their experiences, intentions and desires in words. Some of them give alternative interpretations of everyday reality, lacking intersubjective confirmation. They can act in ways that may be understood as independent and/or irrational or even absurd. In short, people with dementia present behaviour deviating from that of the vast majority of people, and from what is considered to be ideal or desirable for a human being. In this dementia represents 'otherness' or the non-normal. To the extent that dignity has to do with the characteristics of being human, the production and reproduction of dignity is in line with the implementation of the traits of a culturally embraced normality. The maintenance of normality is then in a sense equal to dignity work. Abram De Swaan points out that normality is staged by all the small, everyday things and by the predictability of everyday life:

> Maintaining normality is hard work: a body must be rested, cleaned, groomed, and clothed every day; it must be fed properly and decorously at the correct time and it must be walked on the right tracks and talk the right things. Such normality presupposes that everyone else behaves more or less as expected, and that the entire society pursues its appointed course, so that for any one person the preconditions of achieving his or her individual normality are fulfilled. Society thus enables its members to pursue their business as usual, and at the same time it compels them to do so (De Swaan 1990, p. 1).

At Danneholm the ladies are presented with a culturally guided script telling them what is business as usual, are put on a stage called 'a home' and are instructed in their acting by the staff as the directors. The everyday life of the residential home is guided by the staff, lived under their supervision.

From a cultural perspective, dignity work could be described as a kind of culture work. A simple definition of culture is that it is a set of more or less integrated values, norms and ways of making sense of reality that is irregularly distributed in a collective of human beings sharing similar conditions of living. Culture is continuously being reproduced and more or less transformed (see Hannerz 1992). Presumably, what values constitute dignity of identity vary just as culture varies. In Sweden, as in the Western world as a whole, the individual is for instance seen as a solitary entity that interacts with the environment and other people. This individual is placed in time and space from an understanding of time as linear and with signified distinctions

93

between different points in time and between different places in space. Such cultural understanding of the individual and of time and space interacts with the interpretation of dignity and with how dignity work is done. Discussions on dignity and dignity work could then, and should perhaps always, be considered as explorations and reproductions of culture.

4.7 Summary and concluding remarks on dignity work, normality and power

In this chapter I have focused on dignity of identity work in the everyday life of a residential home designed for people with dementia. The fundamental analytical starting point was that dignity of identity work is produced, reproduced, elaborated and challenged in all the tiny routines, occurrences, acts and deeds of everyday life. Using ethnography from fieldwork in a residential home here given the fictitious name Danneholm, I have outlined and illustrated how the six female residents, called 'the ladies' by the staff, interact with the physical, social and cultural environment in the residential home. Furthermore, I have described the homelike nature of the place and the activities of the staff in reconstructing and upholding the abilities the residents have lost as a consequence of disease. In this way the staff exercise dignity on behalf of the residents. The aim has been to depict what values or ideals constitute dignity, and to describe and analyse the characteristics of dignity of identity work. A secondary aim has been to explore the relation between normality and dignity of identity.

My assertion has been that dignity of identity is constituted by culturally central values. It is impossible to define the concept of dignity without stating some of these values. One central value at Danneholm was that each individual is, or should be, a part of a social context. The ladies were described and deciphered and their life histories reconstructed in the context of former family, relatives and friends. Everyone was expected to be together and enjoy the company of others. This ideal was sometimes challenged by the fact that the ladies couldn't always work out what kind of social gathering they had ended up in. From time to time they became irritated with each other and sometimes got into quarrels which occasionally resulted in mild physical violence.

As a part of a social context a person should exercise autonomy. Autonomy was a cherished ideal at Danneholm. The everyday understanding of autonomy includes the person's ability to be an independent individual with a will of their own, and a capacity to make decisions concerning everyday life. Another culturally central value is a person's sense of the self as a coherent and consistent whole. If the self does not hold up, is experienced as fragmented and irrational, the integrity of identity is in jeopardy. Identity incorporates a life story, and this life story is crucial to the coherence of the self. A person's life is understood as something that can be organised along a timeline, and all the events constituting the story of this life are seen as linked together in a rational and consistent way. At Danneholm much time was dedicated to reconstructing the ladies' life stories. Each resident was 'performed' by the staff as an autonomous individual with a coherent life story that was connected to the here and now of the everyday life of care in the residential home.

Another value, repeatedly expressed at Danneholm, was to be active. The days were filled with different kinds of activities. Some of these related to the running of a house-hold, for instance cleaning, doing laundry, preparing food and washing up. Other activities were the kind of things people usually do at home: having dinner or a cup of coffee together, watching TV or reading the paper. The ladies and the staff celebrated birthdays and the major traditional Swedish festivals. Much time was dedicated to taking care of the ladies' hygiene and appearance. The maintenance of the body could be seen as an expression of another value, that of being clean and tidy and properly dressed. All activities, the maintenance of the body and the celebrations of festivals were ordered into routines. Routines were seen by the staff as a key factor in the care of dementia patients. The routines gave rhythm to the days and the weeks, and orienta-tion in time and space. Routines are a mark of good care and of dignity work. In addi-tion, routines are a cultural value or ideal. This ideal says that a person should be organised and ordered according to time, and do whatever has to be done regularly at the proper hours and on the proper days.

I have stated that the idea of the homelike nature of Danneholm and its staging by the staff could be understood as a kind of summary of all of the cultural values men-tioned above, as well as other values central to dignity of identity. This homelike char-acter is a distillation of well-accepted values and ideals presented to the ladies in the residential home. As discussed, the idea of being homelike is not only an idea of a pleasant environment, it is also an idea of something good and desirable. At the same time, it is a guide and an obligation when it comes to how to present the 'I' and how to act in social interaction. To the ladies, the homelike nature of Danneholm seemed to be a kind of context in which they could feel safe and secure and live an ordinary life. At the same time it was a fragile reality. The ladies could not always decipher whether Danneholm was a home or not, whether it was their home or someone else's home. In this way its homelike character was not only fragile, it could also be a bit confusing.

The staff's performance and reproduction of values – the dignity of identity work done by the staff – could be summarised in four words: reconstruction, surveillance, interpretation and order. They reconstructed the ladies' life stories, the ladies as people and their ability to function socially, as well as an image of 'business as usual' in ordi-nary, everyday home life. This reconstruction, I would suggest, is the more exact meaning of the phrase 'the homelike nature of a residential home for people with dementia'. To keep intact this reconstruction, the homelike nature of Danneholm, they had to be on their guard. Then they could discover if and when the reconstructed reality was about to crack. An important part of this surveillance was to interpret what was going on. The staff constantly interpreted the doings of the ladies in order to suppress and contain disagreement, unease and 'wrong' depictions of reality. Surveillance was accompanied by order. Upholding order was an important tool to prevent flaws in the fragile 'homelike' atmosphere.

While reconstruction, surveillance, interpretation and order were the primary modes of dignity of identity work, the beating heart of the dignity of identity work at Dan-neholm was the message that 'nothing is out of the ordinary'. The homelike nature of the place and the characteristics of the everyday life could be interpreted as indicating that the ladies lived an ordinary life in a normal home where business went on as usual.

This possible interpretation was a bit confusing. The ladies were not really sure about where they were. They constantly tried to work it out, in an ongoing interpretation of the place and what was going on there, an interpretation that never really came to a final conclusion.

The message 'business as usual' and the reproduction of culturally central values could be understood as management of normality. The residential home gave a sense of normality. And, as suggested above, maintaining normality is crucial to the dignity of identity. If someone is regarded and treated as abnormal, as deviant or just a bit different, it may violate their dignity of identity. Whether it does depends on whether that person's identity is founded in some kind of normality or wish to be normal. After all, there are individuals whose identity and dignity are based on being different, not living life as one should according to cultural values and norms. To the extent that dignity of identity is dependent on the ability to maintain normality, the values central to dignity of identity work will be culturally specific. What values are important will vary between different locations of cultural production.

As described in this section, dignity of identity work could be understood as an exercise of power in a Foucauldian sense (Foucault 1990; Bullington, this volume, Chapter 3). Power is then understood as an ongoing process of determining an individual's scope of action and ways of comprehending themselves and the reality they live in. Power is not primarily something someone has and uses against others. Power is exercised by everyone, everywhere and in all kinds of situations. When someone speaks of their dignity in a particular way and tries to act and live this dignity, then that person exercises power. Thus power cannot be seen as simply good or bad. Power is what makes things happen in a certain way. Dignity of identity work presupposes the exercise of power.

The ladies at Danneholm had lost control of everyday decisions about themselves. In other words, to be able to maintain the ladies' dignity the staff had to infringe their autonomy. This was not temporary: the ladies would never regain their autonomy. They were dependent on the staff and on the homelike nature of their environment for exercising autonomy. Still, as the fieldwork examples show, this is not entirely true. Everyday life at Danneholm contained an ongoing struggle of wills and constant negotiation between all the individuals there. The exercise of power presupposes resistance. To make the exercise of power legitimate and meaningful, the resistance has to be interpreted as wrong or bad or a resistance that does not know its own good. This is what happened at Danneholm. At least sometimes, the ladies' own ideas and wills could be taken seriously. If they were not taken seriously, as something threatening the framework of the homelike nature or order of the place, it could just pass, without correction or action. A possible interpretation of this power–resistance relation is that the kind of resistance that does not know its own good was attributed to dementia. Then it was their disease, not the ladies themselves, who resisted the exercise of power aiming at giving autonomy.

According to Nordenfelt (this volume, Chapter 2), dignity of identity has to do with the sense of being an 'integrated and autonomous person'. 'Integrated' could be understood in two senses. One is that a person's identity is tuned into a social whole. This means that the person is a part of one or more social groups (based on e.g. class, ethnicity and sex) and is accepted by significant others as a member, a part of a social interconnectedness. The other meaning of 'integrated' is that the person's identity as such is integrated – that is, the different parts that make up a person's identity are coherent and fit together. Integration of identity in respect of external social belonging and integration of identity in respect of a person's internal coherence of self are dependent on each other. People need to know where they are in space, time and socially to be certain of who they are. And to place yourself in space, time and socially you need to be autonomous. You need to be a separated 'I' in relation to the place you walk in, the time in which you live and the others with whom you interact. Without autonomy it would not be possible to perceive the 'I'. Equally important is the possibility of exercising power over the process of identity. This is another aspect of autonomy: the possibility of exercising power over matters concerning oneself.

This kind of power is of course always more or less formed by the norms, values and routines laid out by others (or by culture or discourse), and it is limited by circumstances outside the control of each individual. Nevertheless, from the individual's point of view they might seem the master of their personal identity. This is a part of autonomy – that is, the idea that one can to at least some extent determine who one is, how one wants to present oneself to others and tell the world 'this is me' and evaluate the world's answer 'this is you as we understand you'. Could a person with dementia be autonomous in this sense? Can people with dementia regard themselves as autonomous in this sense, while the 'normal' people around them do not see them as capable of totally integrating the self?

Probably they can. These questions focus on the individual person's way of comprehending themselves in relation to other humans and to material circumstances. The answer is dependent on a specific person's understanding of what it is to be autonomous – more precisely, on which resources and means, and how much independence of other persons' support, confirmations, desires and needs one requires to imagine oneself as autonomous (see Sandman 2004). The ladies at Danneholm were certainly dependent on the staff for their well-being, and their acts were circumscribed by the needs of other residents and by the necessity to carry on everyday life in the residential home. But still, these ladies all seemed to have very strong preferences and wills. Sometimes they did not consider or respect circumstances and other people, or were not capable of doing so. Now and then they acted as if self-governed, totally independent individuals when singing at the dinner table, proposing a new interpretation of everyday reality, stubbornly holding on to the company of the staff or eating butter directly from the butter dish. Even if a non-demented person would say that this is not normal, it is not how one should behave, it could be that a person suffering from dementia in such situations experiences herself as a person with a high degree of autonomy.

References

Agar, M.H. (1996) *The Professional Stranger: An Informal Introduction to Ethnography*, 2nd edn. Academic Press, San Diego, CA.

de Swaan, A. (1990) *The Management of Normality: Critical Essays in Health and Welfare.* Routledge, London.

Ehn, B. & Löfgren, O. (2001) *Kulturanalyser* [Cultural analysis], 2nd edn. Gleerups, Malmö.

Foucault, M. (1990) *The History of Sexuality*, vol. 1. Random House, New York.

Goffman, E. (1986) *Frame Analysis: An Essay on the Organization of Experience*. Northeastern University Press, Boston, MA.

Goffman, E. (1990) *The Presentation of Self in Everyday Life*. Penguin, London.

Halstead, N. (2001) Ethnographic encounters: positionings within and outside the frame. *Social Anthropology*, **9**, 307–321.

Hannerz, U. (1992) *Cultural Complexity: Studies in the Social Organization of Meaning*. Columbia University Press, New York.

Löfgren, O. (2003) The sweetness of home: class, culture and family life in Sweden. In: *The Anthropology of Space and Place. Locating Culture*, (eds S.M. Low and D. Lawrence-Zúñiga), pp. 142–159. Blackwell, Oxford.

Öhlander, M. (1999) *Skör Verklighet: En Etnologisk Studie av Demensvård i Gruppboende* [A fragile reality. An ethnological study of dementia care in group living], 2nd edn. Studentlitteratur, Lund.

Öhlander, M. (2007) En kulturhistorisk betraktelse av hemmets innebörder [Cultural historical reflections on the meaning of home]. In: *Hemmets Vårdetik: Om Vård av Äldre i Livets Slutskede* [The ethics of home care. On the care of older people at the end of life] (ed. G. Silverberg), pp. 47–65. Studentlitteratur, Lund.

Ortner, S.B. (1973) On key symbols. *American Anthropologist*, **75**, 1338–1346.

Örulv, L. & Nikku, N. (2007) Dignity work in dementia care: sketching a microethical analysis. *Dementia*, **6**, 507–525.

Sandman, L. (2004) On the autonomy-turf: assessing the value of autonomy to patients. *Medicine, Health Care and Philosophy*, **7**, 261–268.

Schatzman, L. & Strauss, A.L. (1973) *Field Research: Strategies for a Natural Sociology*. Prentice-Hall, London.

Schutz, A. (1975) *On Phenomenology and Social Relations. Selected Writings*. University of Chicago Press, Chicago.

5. *Dignity and Older Spouses with Dementia*

Ingrid Hellström

Introduction

One of the most famous life stories in the context of dementia is that of Auguste D, or perhaps, to put it more correctly, Auguste D was Dr Alois Alzheimer's most famous patient. Alois Alzheimer followed and documented the course of Auguste's illness from 1901, when she was admitted to a local psychiatric hospital with agitated behaviour, until 1906 when she died. After her death her brain tissue was examined in detail and her syndrome was later named Alzheimer's disease after her doctor (Page & Fletcher 2006). At that time the focus was on Auguste's individual symptoms and her brain damage. What was crucial was her symptomatic and biological story – not the story of her life in a broader context, nor the story of the joint life with her husband. In this chapter, by contrast, I devote my attention to the stories of husbands and wives living with dementia and my aim is to analyse the notion of dignity in spousal relationships in the context of dementia.

Much of the early work on dementia focused on its biomedical dimensions (Kitwood 1997a) and those studies that explore its impact have tended to focus on the views of family carers, with the overriding emphasis being on understanding caring as a stressful experience (Schulz & Williamson 1997; Montgomery & Williams 2001). However, building on early seminal studies (Hirschfield 1983; Motenko 1989), there is now a growing recognition that caregiving is not a uniformly negative experience and that careers experience satisfaction and rewards (Nolan et al. 1996). Moreover, increasing attention has recently been given to the experiences of people with dementia themselves (Goldsmith 1996; Kitwood 1997a), with Woods (2001) contending that the 'discovery' of personhood in dementia has been one of the most significant recent advances heralding the emergence of a new paradigm of research.

The person with dementia in a social context

Kitwood (1997a, p. 8) uses the concept of personhood, which is 'a standing or status that is bestowed upon one human being, by others, in the context of relationship and social being. It implies recognition, respect and trust'. With Kitwood's concept of personhood social relationships, rather than the person's rational capability, are emphasised. This concept of personhood can be applied to people in later stages of dementia. Dementia should be seen as an interplay between a neurological impairment, the person's mental life and the external events as perceived by the person with dementia. Adopting the idea of personhood in dementia promotes a view of the person with dementia as a social being (Kitwood 1997b). According to Kitwood & Bredin (1992), personhood should be viewed socially. They claim, moreover, that every person has a certain status that is worthy of respect. This status seems to lie close to human dignity or *Menschenwürde*, according to which every living person has an absolute value that is equal among all human beings (Nordenfelt, this volume, Chapter 2).

A general understanding of dementia seems to be that people who have it run the risk of losing their identity and personhood, and that it will lead to total dependency. People with dementia are at great risk of being deprived of dignity. They remain one of the most excluded groups in Western society, being subjected to the deleterious effects of two powerful stigmas: ageing and increasing cognitive frailty (Dewing 2002; Wilkinson 2002). Cotrell & Schultz (1993) differentiate between two forms of stigma: felt and enacted stigma. *Felt stigma* is the person's own experienced shame at having a particular illness, for example Alzheimer's disease. *Enacted stigma*, on the other hand, is the discrimination due to the person's Alzheimer's disease.

Post (1995, p. 3) states that:

Rather than allowing declining mental capacities to divide humanity into those who are worthy or unworthy of full moral attention, it is better to develop an ethics based on the essential unity of human beings and on an assertion of equality despite unlikeness of mind.

We live in a hypercognitive culture (Post 1995) and there is a division between '*us* (members of the "normal" population) and *them* (the dementia sufferers)' (Kitwood & Bredin 1992, p. 272). Calnan & Tadd (this volume, Chapter 6) write that one of the most horrifying prospects of the future for many older Europeans is to be stricken with dementia in old age, and there is a general understanding that dementia is inevitably accompanied by loss of identity and personhood and increasing dependency. There are negative images of ageing and old age in Western society, and the notion of senility (dementia) has contributed to a great extent to this understanding. In everyday language, senility is used in the sense of decline due to old age. It seems that the negative images developed during the 19th century when there was an interest in describing ageing and old age systematically in the medical literature (Kirk 1995; Swane 1996). Every society has central cultural values and these are interlinked with a person's identity (Öhlander, this volume, Chapter 4). The 'attribute' dementia (senility) has a low value in a hypercognitive society and this low value influences the dignity of a person with dementia.

According to Nordenfelt (this volume, Chapter 2) the dignity of identity relates to a person's integrity, autonomy, life history and relationships with others. This dignity – unlike human dignity or *Menschenwürde* – may vary depending on the attitude of others towards an individual, and is consequently influenced by changes to an individual's body and mind. People may be looked down upon if they have a decreased ability to act autonomously, or lack certain capacities and endowments. Older people with dementia are at risk of losing such dignity. We think that people with dementia (*them*) constitute a problem, without seeing that the problem could be located within *us* (Kitwood & Bredin 1992).

100

Sabat (2001, 2002) points out that we must distinguish between how the identity of a person appears to others, and how that person experiences and expresses their own identity. He differentiates between three selves: the self of personal identity (Self 1), the self of mental and physical attributes and beliefs about those attributes (Self 2), and the socially presented self (Self 3). A person's experience of their personal identity is expressed specifically through the use of first-person pronouns such as *I, me*. What the person is with respect to Self 2 (e.g. religious orientation, sense of humour, good memory and eyesight) can vary over time, and some attributes are more easily affected than others. Self 3 is dependent on the social context within which one finds oneself, and requires interplay with at least one other person. Therefore a person with dementia is vulnerable and dependent on other persons in social situations. Sabat (2002) argues that a loss of Self 3 need not be dependent chiefly on the brain damage caused by dementia but instead on a lack of support from others in the person's social world.

The three selves are also important with respect to who is describing a person. A person's life story is an important and well-known aid in dementia care. Lantz (this volume, Chapter 8), however, argues that the telling itself has an aspect of power, and an impact on a person's identity. The story of a person's life is dependent on who is telling it. Lantz differentiates between first-, second- and third-person telling. In first-person telling the person narrates their own life story, and has the power or control over how it is presented. In third-person telling, another person tells the story and has the power, for example, to define a person's character. A person with dementia could be described as clinging because they are afraid of being alone. The lives of people with dementia are often reconstructed 'with fragments of life stories' (Öhlander, this volume, Chapter 4), and third-person telling is often used in such a context. Second-person telling takes the form of a dialogue and in the interaction life stories appear (Lantz, this volume, Chapter 8). Second-person telling can be used to uphold Self 3 (Sabat 2001), which is dependent on social interaction with at least one other person.

Nordenfelt (this volume, Chapter 2) presents a special kind of dignity attached to older people: the dignity of wisdom, which he considers to be a species of dignity of merit. Wisdom in this sense is not knowledge of facts, but a combination of the knowledge of human beings and an attitude towards them. Older people have lived a long time and have had a multitude of experiences. Admittedly, individual older people are wise to different degrees. Nordenfelt argues, however, that the dignity of wisdom can be ascribed to older people as a group. A second special merit which is attached to older people is that of their achievements and efforts. Older people have, for example, put in an intensive effort for society and for their families. We should pay respect to their achievements and listen to their experiences and advice.

We may then ask: how do we support the older people with dementia so that they can live well, and how do we uphold their dignity of wisdom and their dignity of achievement and effort? There is a great risk that our knowledge about them will be very limited. For example, until recently people with dementia were excluded from research and our understanding of the experience of dementia was based on proxy accounts provided primarily by family carers (Bamford & Bruce 2000; Bond & Corner 2001). Moreover, our understanding of the subjective experience of people with dementia is mostly based on interviews with people who have mild to moderate dementia.

Thus there is a need for research to understand the subjective experience of people with more severe dementia (O'Connor et al. 2007).

The concepts of personhood and person-centred care (Kitwood 1997a; Nolan et al. 2002) are highly influential in both policy and practice, not only in dementia care but also in a wide range of other care settings. Furthermore, the relationship between the person with dementia and others, particularly the family carer(s), is now seen as a key factor in maintaining a sense of self and personhood for the person (Crisp 1999; Whitlach 2001; Phinney 2002). However, relatively few studies have focused on the nature of such relationships (see, for example, Sällström 1994; Perry 1995; Keady 1999; Kaplan 2001), particularly as experienced by both parties (Forbat 2003). Consequently, there is a need to explore how a person's subjective experiences of dementia are shaped within the context of personal relationships, both from the viewpoint of the person with dementia and from the viewpoint of others. Dementia in the context of a spousal relationship, the specific focus of this chapter, is geared to such a double analysis.

Spouses living with dementia

Corbin & Strauss (1988) note that an appreciation of the nature of dyadic relationships is essential to a full understanding of the way in which people adjust to chronic illnesses more generally. They advocate that a temporal perspective should be adopted, and their study identified the differing types of 'work' that people with a chronic illness and their spouses engage in over time. 'Work' is defined as 'a set of tasks performed by an individual or a couple, alone or in conjunction with others, to carry out a plan of action designed to manage one or more aspects of the illness and the lives of ill people and their partners' (Corbin & Strauss 1988, p. 9). It is significant that the couple's illness management is part of their ongoing life. Corbin & Strauss (1988) also differentiate between the illness trajectory and the course of illness. The *course of illness* is described in biomedical terms, e.g. each dementia diagnosis has its own predetermined route. On the other hand, the *illness trajectory* is each couple's unique accommodation to a chronic illness, and the impact of the illness on their daily life and the 'work' that is needed. Corbin & Strauss (1988) place considerable emphasis on biographical work, i.e. people's efforts to redefine and reintegrate their biographical identity in the face of chronic illness, together with their carers. The authors indicate that the emotional elements of biographical work are the most demanding.

Few studies have focused on the relationship between people with dementia and their carers (Forbat 2003). However, the limited work conducted to date suggests that multidimensional and dynamic interrelationships between people with dementia and their carers exist throughout the experience of dementia (Whitlach 2001). This reinforces the fact that to consider the person with dementia as an 'interdependent subject' does not tell the whole story, and that it is also important to recognise the possibility that their being is 'constituted through being in relation to others' (Phinney 2002). This suggests that there is much to be gained by paying attention to the 'dynamic interrelationships' noted above (Whitlach 2001). One of the most detailed accounts of the dynamic nature of relationships between people with dementia and their carers is provided by Keady (1999), who interviewed both the family carer and the person with dementia, asking them to recount their earliest recollections of the disease from when they first noticed that something was amiss, up until the point of formal diagnosis and beyond.

Keady elaborated upon Corbin & Strauss' (1988) concept of 'work in chronic illness'. According to Keady (1999), in most caring relationships the main motivation of the non-affected spouse throughout the process of working was to 'maintain the involvement' of the person with dementia by creating ways in which their sense of agency and self could be sustained for as long as possible.

The dynamics of 'couplehood' in dementia

This chapter is mainly based on a longitudinal interview study of 20 older people with dementia and their spouses (Hellström 2005; Hellström et al. 2007). The aim of the study was to explore the ways in which older people with dementia and their spouses experience dementia over time, especially the impact it has on their interpersonal relationships and patterns of everyday life. At inclusion the spouses were 65–85 years old. They had been living together for between 8 and 60 years, most of them for over 50 years. Initially, two researchers interviewed the spouses separately and simultaneously in different rooms, but at the end of the study joint interviews were more common. Over 150 interviews with the couples were conducted on five or six occasions during the period 2001–2006, involving both spouses. The interviews were structured around the following themes: the home, memory disturbance, quality of everyday life and their relationship, and dignity and autonomy. Three interviews were conducted with staff caring for three study participants, two at a day-care centre and one at a residential home.

An analysis of the complete data set identified three temporally sequenced but overlapping phases: sustaining couplehood, maintaining involvement (after Keady 1999) and moving on (Table 5.1).

Sustaining couplehood captures the efforts made by both spouses to maintain, and where possible enhance, the quality of their lives together for as long as possible, and this was the ultimate aim of the couples' 'work'. This involved four interrelated sets of activities: talking things through, in order to ensure good communication and acknowledge and value differences; being affectionate and appreciative by demonstrating continued attraction to their spouse; making the most of things by enjoying everyday

Table 5.1 Phases in the experience of dementia

Sustaining couplehood	Talking things through Being affectionate and appreciative Making the best of things Keeping the peace
Maintaining involvement	Playing an active part Taking risks Handing over Letting go Taking over
Moving on	Remaining a 'we' Becoming an 'I' New beginning

pleasures, looking for positive interpretations of events and focusing on the present; and finally, keeping the peace by being aware of potential points of friction and not responding to difficult behaviour. Both the person with dementia and the non-affected spouse were active strategists in the above process. The following quotation is from a husband who tries to look for positive interpretations of their present life together:

Of course it's sad to live together with a person who is one's life companion to see how she changes. Yes, because we have had a good life before. It's totally changed. It's not funny. Then you have to find the positive things in life. You always search for the positive to be able to feel happy. You can't go and dig yourself in, you have to find new angles, which make it more positive.

Sustaining couplehood and maintaining involvement are not linear phases, with one preceding the other. Rather, as emerged in the earlier interviews, the two processes occurred simultaneously, with sometimes one, sometimes the other, being the major focus of attention. Here is one example of how the couples 'do things together' in order to take care of the domestic routine:

I mean, it works very well. She [wife with dementia] does laundry and ironing, we clean together. I vacuum and she dusts, so it works well, and then we go shopping together as much as we can, otherwise I go myself. It depends on how much she has got to do at home.

In addition both spouses worked to 'maintain involvement' of the person with dementia by ensuring that they had an active role to play. However, despite their efforts, the non-affected spouse eventually took on an increasing role in one of two ways: either by the person with dementia consciously handing over responsibility or more passively letting go, or by the non-affected spouse taking over. Sometimes maintaining an active involvement of the spouse with dementia meant taking quite a high degree of risk, as for example where one person with dementia wanted to continue his established routine of going into town alone on the bus.

At the end of the study, despite their best efforts to maintain involvement and sustain couplehood, the spouses were increasingly 'working alone' (Keady 1999) and had begun to feel alone. A husband described their situation at home like this:

Yes, despite the fact that we are living together, and we have got a lot in common, nevertheless we are lonely in a way. I do my things, sitting at the computer or out working, and she is in here pottering. Staring at TV, mostly sitting sleeping. You live in two small worlds. You have a common world and then you have your own world besides.

By the time of the follow-up interviews with 11 couples in 2005–2006, this process had progressed and things had moved on. Six couples were still living at home, three of the people with dementia had gone into residential care and two had recently died. From the analysis of the data, three couples were still maintaining involvement with the active input by the spouse with dementia. Four couples remained a 'we', where the focus of their efforts was on the couple rather on the individual, albeit with the spouse with dementia now playing a far less active role. In the cases where the person with dementia had gone into residential care one spouse still defined themself as being a part of a couple, and took an active pleasure in the company of the person with dementia, e.g. through going walking. Elements of being affectionate and making the best of things were therefore still evident, but now with a more passive role on the part of the person with dementia. One spouse was still making an effort to remain a 'we', but was increasingly becoming an 'I', no longer defining themself as part of a couple. In another case, the wife's admission to residential care, and her increasing aggression, meant that the husband involved was becoming an 'I' and starting to forge a new beginning for himself without his wife. In the two instances where the person with dementia had died, one spouse still defined herself very closely as part of a couple and found it difficult to move on to a new beginning, whereas the other, while still retaining fond memories of her spouse, had begun to create a new life for herself.

In the following section, the notion of dignity in spousal relationships will be analysed. The data are based on the interviews with the 11 couples who participated in the study at 5–6 points in time during 2001–2006.

5.1 Dignity in spousal relationships

The description of the notion of dignity takes its starting point in the quotation below. Robert, who had Alzheimer's disease, lived in a beautiful flat with his wife Maria, whom he had married almost 50 years ago. They seemed to have a very good marital relationship and a good relationship with their four children. He had been a successful businessman and had been very active in different business associations. In the first and second interviews we talked about whether Robert still felt that other people respected him as before. He thought they did, but he also had impaired hearing and in the second interview he said that these two handicaps 'created a new human being'. He felt like a new human being, partly because he was not able to participate in his associations as before, because of his two handicaps. During the third interview with Robert the concept of dignity was brought up explicitly once more. He gave a very rich answer that seemed to cover several important aspects of dignity that were brought up during the interviews with the 11 participating couples. Henceforth the description will be structured around the quotation below.

> Interviewer (I): *Then* [in the last interview] *we also talked about dignity, if a person's dignity alters when one gets a disease. How do you look at it today?*
> Robert: *Yes, I think it's a little different in different stages* [of the disease]. *The pure notion of dignity, I think it should not need to be influenced by any disease. It depends on how other people look upon the person who is ill. People are often a little ruthless, and value people around them differently depending on their competence in one way or another. Here we, as human beings, are a little poor. But our strong wish is that it should be this way, that the relations within and outside the family need not change too much because one family member is ill.*

Robert pointed out how important it is that a person who is ill should not be regarded as of less value than other people. He has the same absolute value as a human being that anyone else has, his human dignity or *Menschenwürde* (Nordenfelt, this volume,

Chapter 2). However, Robert also saw his disease in different stages and how this could influence the dignity of a person.

5.1.1 The disease has different stages

Robert thought that a person's dignity could alter when they get a disease, and the alteration depends on what stage of the disease they are in.

The participants in the interview study were aware that they had a disease which would get worse over time, and they could see that other people with the disease were more fragile and also that this could be their situation in the future, with no connection with reality as we know it, and with increasing dependence on other people. They felt that their disease had a specific, and often predetermined, course (Corbin & Strauss 1988). One man with Alzheimer's disease talked about what his diagnosis could mean for him in the future. He explicitly used the term 'vegetable':

> *But, obviously it's a sad development to become a vegetable. That you don't wish for, of course. But you don't have much of a choice.*

When he talked about an ordinary day he said that he used to take a stroll in the nearby park on his own. His wife had difficulty in accompanying him because of pain in her hip. He knew that there was a risk of his becoming disoriented and getting lost during his walk. He also talked about one of his friends who once been lost in town, dressed only in his pyjamas. He said that he had not experienced that, not yet anyway, but he knew it was possible that it could happen to him in the near future.

Several of the people with dementia who participated in the study experienced speech impairment. They thought that this affected their identity and thereby their dignity. A person's dignity of identity can be influenced by their illness (Nordenfelt, this volume, Chapter 2). One man described in the interview how he felt when he started to lose his voice. He felt that his voice was very weak and he had also lost words and names of people he knew very well. This was very humiliating, as he thought that when the voice is gone, the person is gone.

> I: *Is there something you think could humiliate you?*
> PWD: *Yes, I suppose if I lose my voice. Then you disappear entirely.*
> I: *If you can't express yourself?*
> PWD: *Yes, lose words and so on, if you see a face and look the picture of bewilderment.*

His wife was well aware of this and was very careful to help him join in conversations. She had some experience from a friend who cared for his wife with dementia and never let his wife answer for herself. She thought that it was important to let her husband talk himself, and this was a part of his dignity.

> *I will not do that with my husband, he has to answer himself, as long as he is capable of it, and then I don't know if it will become too difficult over time. In most cases I notice it's me who is talking and talking, but I really want him to join in, because I want an answer from him 'Isn't that so? Eh?' Eventually it's too much for him and he has to answer.*

The wife thought the speech impairment would 'become too difficult' and then she would have to take over for him completely. The wife adjusted to her husband's 'illness trajectory' (Corbin & Strauss 1988). Another man with dementia experienced the same problem. He had been very active in different associations and he and his wife used to do folk dancing together. During the period of the study he had started to withdraw from these activities because of his difficulty in expressing himself. He said that he could not express himself and this deficit had an effect on his self-respect.

I: *So your value as a person has changed since you got memory problems?*
PWD: *I suppose it's myself, eh, I just stand there babbling sometimes, I can't express what I want to say, and that makes you feel small, you might say, that you can't express yourself.*
I: *Is it more your own view, that the self-respect is changing?*
PWD: *Yes, it is that, I think, as a matter of fact.*

At the time of the last interview he was living in residential care and it was almost impossible to interpret his utterances. His wife had to speak for him.

Some people with dementia in the interview study compared themselves with older and frailer people they were acquainted with. One woman with early Alzheimer's disease told me about the 'old ladies' at the charity shop where she used to help out. She was humiliated when her older friends pointed out that she forgot things they had told her about in the shop. She returned to this several times during the interviews and she repeated the sentence 'I told you a long time ago', almost word for word each time. Repeated sentences are often interpreted as a symptom of dementia; the person has difficulty in remembering what they narrated earlier. The sentence could also be interpreted in the perspective of a first-person narration (Lantz, this volume, Chapter 8): the woman narrated something that was very important to her, which she expressed through her story (Swane 1996). In spite of the fact that she was humiliated by this sentence she tried to ignore it and did not comment on it in front of her friends. She thought that one should take the fact that they were older than she was into consideration. She simply ignored that they also forget things.

PWD: *But I do get sad when one of my friends says '****I told you that a long time ago****' (emphasis added). Sometimes they can be a little mean, old ladies, there are a lot of old people* [at the charity shop] *you know, whom I have known for several years.*
I: *In what way are they mean, then?*
PWD: *They just say something, you know 'No, but ****I told you that a long time ago!****' (emphasis added), or 'Don't you remember that?' or something like that. On the whole they are nice people so that's nothing, but they are much older than me, you know, so I notice that they are a little gaga* [laughing].

She made a distinction between the people who were older and a 'little gaga', and people like herself who just had certain problems in daily life.

The spouses wanted to live together as long as possible, but they knew that if the dementia got a lot worse the person with dementia would have to move to sheltered accommodation. One woman with Alzheimer's disease was afraid of ending up in a nursing home. She was very pleased that her husband was able to help her so that she could still live in their home.

PWD: *It would have been humiliating, no I don't want that.*
I: *At another place, what do you mean by that?*
PWD: *I don't know where they could think of sending me, putting me in, then.*
I: *Sheltered housing, you mean then?*
PWD: *Yes.*
I: *It's what you are thinking of, then?*
PWD: *Yes, an institution or something like that. I want to be at home, we have a nice time together.*

Another woman said that if she ended up in a nursing home, her independence and autonomy would be affected. She used to visit a close friend, who was living in the nursing home in the village, once a week. Her own mother had lived in the same nursing home and she thought that the life there was quite different from her life in her own home. During the interviews she often came back to the fact that she was delighted still to be able to walk around her house and look at all her things and furniture. She said that all her furniture had a history to tell. In a nursing home she would lose this possibility of walking around her house and garden. It seemed that both women talked about and identified themselves with their homes and spousal relationships. The woman cited in the quotation above clearly connected life at 'an institution' with degradation of her dignity of identity.

The spouses were, of course, also aware that their partner had a disease that was expected to get worse over time. One frequent apprehension among the spouses was that they had to live longer than their wife/husband with dementia, and they also wanted to help them as long as they possibly could. The main reason was that they wanted to stay together. Another reason was that they could guarantee more dignified care. If possible, most of them did not want to place their spouse in a residential home:

And that day I hope to be living at least, we have talked about it, who is going to die first, and now I hope I will manage to take care of my husband for as long as possible, because I intend to, I don't want to send him anywhere, that worries me.

One wife had a bad experience of a care home where her mother had lived. She thought they provided undignified care and gave several examples of why she thought so. One example was that on several occasions she had found her mother sitting with a wet nappy. She did not want to let this happen to her own husband. So one distinct pattern among the spouses was that they wanted to live longer than their partner with dementia; they wanted to be there for them. One husband said during the interview that he was very careful with his health and used to jog several times a week. He also had to give up his great interest in motor sport. He was not afraid for his own safety, but he knew that his wife needed his support for at least a few years more. Below is a quotation from a wife who took care of her husband with Alzheimer's disease. She had problems with her heart, and she was worried that she might have a heart attack. Her husband was aware of her illness and he used to check up, for example if she had been staying in the toilet to long.

> I: *Are you worried that something is going to happen to your health?*
> Wife: *I don't worry about myself, but I want to live long enough that my husband doesn't suffer. It's the only thing.*
> I: *Have you talked about this risk?*
> Wife: *No, we always hope to be together. That is what we say every night. 'I can't manage without you', he tells me. He is incredibly thankful for whatever I do. I don't want him to feel he's a burden to me. Instead I always try to cover up.*

The study participants, both the people with dementia and the spouses, were aware of the impact of dementia on their everyday life, but most of them reached a conscious decision not to dwell upon the implications of this but rather to focus on the present and to make life as meaningful and enjoyable as possible.

5.1.2 People with dementia are looked on in different ways

Robert said in the introductory quotation that dignity is dependent on 'how other people look upon the person who is ill' and he added that 'people are often a little ruthless'.

People with dementia run the risk of being treated as objects, not as subjects, especially if the people around them do not acknowledge their problems in daily life or do not have enough knowledge about the disease. One study participant, a man with mixed dementia, had great problems with orientation in time. He had trouble remembering how old he was, but he knew very well that he was born in 1922. He needed physiotherapy after an accident, and for a time he attended day care. He was not so keen on the exercise programmes; he preferred to sit and talk to the other participants in the group and to the staff, and to share his life story. According to his wife, some of the staff paid no consideration to the fact that his time orientation was badly affected by his disease. They rather made a joke of his problems. His wife told of an incident at the day-care centre. Her husband was very keen on talking about his life. However, his stories were mixed up in time. He had owned a dog and it had run away a couple of times. He told the group that he had lost his dog. When his wife arrived at the day-care centre, one of the staff asked about the lost dog. She told him that the dog had died a long time ago and that her husband sometimes tended to forget it. Next time at the day-care centre, the man told the group about his walking trips in the mountains of northern Sweden. He had led groups several times and had been very competent in this area. At this point the nursing assistant who was leading the group ridiculed him, and told him that he had made up a fairy tale. There was no understanding that a person could talk about different stages in their life at the same time. The staff did not acknowledge his achievements and efforts, and this form of dignity of merit was neglected.

One other study participant with dementia had difficulty in distinguishing the programmes on TV from the room he and his wife were sitting in. This could sometimes make watching TV very stressful for him. This quotation describes one episode when they were watching a cookery programme:

Wife: *So after that episode he doesn't want to see the programme if he can't eat any of the food [in the programme]. If I ask him if he's hungry and wants a sandwich, he just says 'I'm not hungry, I don't need any food'.*
I: *So he got nothing when the cook served the others on the television?*
Wife: *Yes, some weeks ago when we were watching the TV cook he said 'We can go to her', and he got up. But I told him that she was on TV. 'We'll just walk around the corner and then we'll come to her', he said. He believes in the TV.*

His wife was able to interpret his feelings for the TV. Unfortunately this perception of TV continued when he moved to the residential home. The staff did not acknowledge his feelings for the TV; they just thought he spoiled the evening for the other residents. This short excerpt is from an interview with an nursing assistant at his group home.

Member of staff (M): *He places himself in front of the TV, like this, in order to stop the others from seeing the TV screen. And he has a conversation with the TV, you see.*
I: *Yes, he does.*
M: *It's very real for him.*
I: *But it's nothing he's afraid of?*
M: *I don't think so, no. On the other hand, we have noticed that he becomes more and more aggressive.*
I: *How does it show?*
M: *For one thing, he becomes upset, you see, he just shakes.*
I: *Mm.*
M: *But then he tries to hit out.*

This example shows how vulnerable and dependent a person with dementia can be in a social situation. The person's social self (Sabat 2001) would not have been presented as 'aggressive' in this situation if he had had the right support from persons around him. The way people act towards a person with dementia has a great influence on the individual's well-being. Through pure thoughtlessness or ignorance, people can behave ruthlessly, as Robert put it.

5.1.3 I still matter
Let us go back to Robert's utterance for a third time. He said that people are valued 'depending on their competence in one way or another'.

Most people have an important position in a social context; people with dementia are no exception. The participants in the study were or had been engaged in several important activities in society, but most of their achievements were in the past. One woman had recently retired when she was diagnosed as having Alzheimer's disease. She had held different positions in the local church that were important to her. Her father had been a churchwarden, and both she and her husband had the same position in the church. For a long time she had also helped the lay worker visiting older people in the neighbourhood and running group activities for children.

At the beginning of the study she still held her position as a churchwarden, but the clergyman had adapted her duties to her altered functions in daily life. For example, he gave her an easier text to read during the service. But after a time these adaptations did not help her as much as she had hoped, so she started to feel more and more afraid of making mistakes during the service, and resigned her position as churchwarden.

> PWD: *Yes, if I forgot something, you know, and you think when you are in church among people it's a bit awkward like that, no but my husband, he's still going to the church* [as churchwarden], *so at that time it was both of us.*
> I: *So this with the church, it was you, not anyone else ...?*
> PWD: *No, no, it wasn't. I felt it myself, because if you have that position, it's a bit, it has to be right, yes, yes, you can forget, one never knows.*

She was afraid that she would forget important things in front of the congregation, so she resigned her position. Nevertheless she did not seem to attribute any great importance to this fact; she thought she still had a position in the community by being able to help at the church café and church choir practice every Tuesday. After a while she also started to attend a day-care centre for people with dementia, and there she used her experiences from the church to help other guests at the centre. I visited her once at the centre. It was close to Christmas and the guests were preparing different articles for a Christmas market they were organising for their families. It was obvious that she and another woman were leading the work for the market. She could use all her remaining skills in a safer context, with no risk of losing face.

One man with mixed dementia had lost the faculty of speech, and the follow-up interview was conducted as a joint interview. Earlier he had said that the ability to speak was very important for dignity. His wife was aware of his feelings and explained to him that he had a disease, just as she had problems with her hip and could not walk properly. And she often comforted him by saying: 'It's so good that you run errands for me and I think for you'. She was also very careful to call attention to his former position as an engineer and to his many business journeys to Japan and the USA. She had made an album where she had written down all his trips to help him to remember them, and so the other members of his family could read about his achievements in his professional life.

> I: *This file, is it something you have made yourself that he should read?*
> Wife: *It was when we went through* [the papers] *and had to throw away so much, then he said 'My trips to America, we won't chuck away these papers'. 'No we won't', I said. ... We started to talk, suddenly things pop up, things he remembers, that he had been to the USA and then it crossed my mind that I should write down all his trips.*

During the progression of dementia the person was losing different talents and knowledge.

In the study it was common for the spouses to talk about their partner's talents, some of which they were not able to exercise any more. One man with Alzheimer's disease had been very good at maths and had worked as an engineer, but he lost his ability to handle the domestic accounts during his illness. In the early 1970s it was he who had planned the estate they lived in. His wife compared the present and the past, and his

111

loss of mathematical skills had had an influence on her too. She thought it was hard to see him struggling.

> I: *You told me he has difficulty in counting, so have you taken over those sorts of things?*
> Wife: *No, it might be that I have to write, what is it called, we have a postal giro bank account, so you know you have to write everything and add up the figures, and you have to write that carefully, the giro number, and that is difficult for him. I have to check and sometimes he hasn't really managed and made a mistake. Sometimes he hasn't added up the figures correctly, but it is very difficult with figures, so he can't do that any more, and it is horrible to see, you wouldn't believe it, but that's how it is.*
> I: *Do you think he is aware of this himself?*
> Wife: *Yes he does … he notices as well, more than he admits to me, I understand that, and I have not shown him that I am sad, I haven't, at least I have tried. It has happened sometimes that I have shown him anyway, but I don't want to.*

People in the later stages of dementia are often dependent on others to tell their life story. In the case of one participating couple, the wife brought up the subject. She knew that she was the only one who could tell her husband's life story. They had no children, and all his close relatives were dead. The husband was confined to a wheelchair as a result of an accident and he had major problems with his memory, especially orientation in time. Often it was hard for him to remember how old he was and if he had to go to work in the morning. The wife emphasised that he had been a very strong man and he had built most of the house they were living in. He had been a good driver, and they had been on several car trips in Europe on holiday. He had also led walking tours in the mountains of northern Sweden. As his dementia got worse he started to be afraid of a lot of things: heights, going by car, violence in TV programmes and so on. But she always tried to call attention to his former achievements, his former identity.

5.1.4 Relations with other people
Finally, I will turn to Robert's own utterances about dignity. He wished that 'the relations within and outside should not change too much because one member of the family is ill'.

How do the spouses handle the relations within and outside the spousal relationship? One wife thought it was important to maintain her husband's remaining skills as long as possible. However, she said it was like a balancing act. Sometimes she had to point out for him that he had done something wrong, but most of the time she restrained herself in order not to harm his self-esteem.

> Wife: *It's obvious that it's not funny all the time to learn that you are not good, or not doing the right thing … but I'm working on it* [laughing], *yes, no I'm working hard, I try to constrain myself, but I have to say that I'm not always handling it, so sometimes it's like before: 'Why have you done that?' So it's like that.*
> I: *Do you regret it afterwards?*

Wife: *Yes, I regret it, and then I go and try to be nice again, but it's obvious you don't want to be mean, that you don't want, but it's hard, it's very hard, the balancing act, it's like walking a tightrope.*

She tried as long as possible to keep her husband with dementia involved in everyday life, but at the same time the domestic routines have to function, for instance they have to pay their monthly bills.

One husband was well aware of his wife's problems with regard to handling different things in everyday life. She was diagnosed as having Alzheimer's disease. She had been employed as a clerk and she used to handle all the financial matters at home. He acknowledged her interest in keeping up to date with household financial affairs. He organised the bills and so on in such a way that she could handle them. But eventually he had to take over all of this work because she became too agitated.

And to handle financial matters and like that, it's too hard for her. It's just as well, bills and things like that I handle myself. Generally speaking I do it when she's not at home, because if she's at home she makes a mess of all the papers and spreads them all over the table.

He showed consideration for his wife by doing this work when she was at a day-care centre so she should be spared the frustration of not managing to cope with it. He did not want to humiliate her by letting her try.

One man with Alzheimer's disease had earlier taken part in different associations. During the interview he felt that he did not have the same benefit from the meetings as he had before. And he also felt vulnerable because he could not follow the discussions as before. He withdrew from the meetings in order not to expose himself.

I: *You said that you do not need to take part in every meeting and things like that. Is it a way to protect oneself as a person, not to expose oneself? Do I understand you correctly, then?*
PWD: *Yes, it can contribute to whether you want to go or not. If you know, or are pretty sure, that you will be unpleasantly affected, it's nice if you don't need to go.*

His wife experienced this as a great loss, both for herself and for her husband. She thought that he had no reason to hide from their friends. His friends were old and frail too, and there was no need to feel ashamed. She expressed no felt stigma (Cotrell & Schultz 1993) in relation to her husband's dementia, but he did.

I: *Last time, you said that the social relations are a bit restricted.*
Wife: *Yes they are, but we pull some strings here so we have been seeing each other a little bit more nowadays. Then you notice that everyone has their own problems. We are in the same boat, and we joke about everything. We needn't be ashamed if we feel a little stupid one way or another, you have to take it as it is. Sooner or later it will come to the surface for everyone.*

At one interview session we began a joint interview with a woman with dementia and her husband. She had made the coffee and poured it out. After a short while she

113

offered us another cup, which we accepted. When she went to the kitchen her husband bent forward and told us in a low voice, 'I know the coffee is weak, but I would never tell her that'. His wife had been a matron at a boarding school and managing her household had great importance for her, but sometimes she made mistakes; nevertheless her husband would never point it out to her. Over time her husband had to take over the cooking, and she was very sorry about that. This is an excerpt from a joint interview.

I: *It's you* [husband] *who cook nowadays?*
Husband: *Yes … it's a little hard for her to keep check on the spices so sometimes …*
PWD: *It's crazy, you see.*
Husband: *Yes, you know …*
PWD: *Can't believe you can be like this, my memory has been so good.*

She also started to get lost outside their house. She did not always agree with her husband that she had problems with her orientation. She felt like a 'prisoner' when he had advised her not to go out on her own. She did not feel trusted at all. Her husband also knew that she had problems with regard to participating in different activities at their church and he was very careful to help her out and explain different things for her so she could take part. It was very important that she should not feel alone.

I: *Does everyone* [at the church] *know about her problems?*
Husband: *Yes, most of them. As I say, it's nothing to conceal because when they talk to her they notice she says the same thing several times. … It will not turn out better if you do not talk about it. I say how it is. I'm doing all right, although I have to help her and I do it with pleasure. So when we are out we always sit down together, and it happens that I need to help her with something and she wants me to, she feels alone otherwise.*

The last example is about a woman with dementia who had worked for a charitable organisation for a long time. The first time we met, this assignment was very important to her. She talked a lot about her achievements for the organisation and she identified herself with the work in the charity shop. And she said 'I gladly participate down there and work from time to time'. However, she acknowledged her bad memory and said that she tried her best to remember everything around her but then it just disappeared. She also experienced difficulty in following when several people talked at the same time, and it was hard for her to take in new information. She said in the first interview that there was a lot of talking in the shop. According to her husband she had earlier been the 'leading lady' in the organisation. He was also active in the organisation and helped out with the financial side. But he gave another perspective on their work at the charity shop. In the interviews he said that the shop had dominated their life for a long time and he thought that the other members did not take his wife seriously after they had learnt she was diagnosed as having Alzheimer's disease.

The other ladies notice it and they want to put her aside in a way, and then I get annoyed of course, because they don't take her seriously and that is almost the worst thing I would say, the way they do it, since all her life revolves around this charity shop. She constantly talks about it, so it's almost the most important thing she has.

Over time she started to feel insecure about her achievement in the shop, and she said that the shop was not that important any more. It was more important to let the younger members of the organisation do their bit. However, she still helped her husband with the financial side.

I can do it and if I want to come down and work I'm allowed to. But the staff have changed one by one. Some are old and don't want to volunteer any longer, and I can understand them. They can't manage. I have been working with the charity shop for so many years so I think I have done my bit now. But I enjoyed the time when I was working all the time, actually.

At the fourth interview with the couple she had stopped volunteering at the shop. And the husband concluded:

We were active in the charity shop a lot before, but she has left it completely now. She doesn't want to hear about it. It is the security she wants, I suppose. I want to enjoy life in a way, to eat will and to feel good and so on.

To sum up, both spouses were well aware that the dementia probably would get worse over time, and this could have an influence on dignity, especially if the voice faded away or if the spouse with dementia was not able to live at home any longer. The couples' stories also show that the people with dementia are vulnerable and their well-being is dependent on how other people act towards them and how they interact with them. However, the people with dementia still had important roles in society despite their illness, albeit some achievements were in the past.

5.2   Conclusions

People with dementia are dependent on social relations to uphold their personhood (Kitwood 1997a), and it seems that the analysis of dignity in most of the literature is based on the individual person. This raises a problem when applying the notion in the context of dementia.

Holm (2001) uses the metaphor of Neurath's boat, which was originally a description of science, to illustrate what is happening to a person with dementia over time:

Whereas the normal person gradually exchanges old planks in her boat of knowledge and personality for new ones while sailing on the sea of life, the person with progressive dementia is steadily losing planks without any replacements. Initially the shape of the boat stays the same, but as time goes by it disintegrates into smaller and smaller pieces, each floating separately in a sea of lost memories (Holm 2001, p. 153).

But is it possible to be a lonely sailor on the sea of life? People with dementia need support to 'replace planks' during the illness trajectory, or at least careful help in reconstructing their life story and their identity. In a spousal relationship, both members of a couple 'sail the boat' and over time it is the spouse who is cognitively intact becomes increasingly more responsible for the 'shape of the boat', their common life story and their co-constructed dignity. Dignity seems to be interrelated between the two members of the couple; humiliation of one spouse often means humiliation of the couple. In the spouses' descriptions of dignity there is no doubt that both in the couple accommodate (Corbin & Strauss 1988) to the illness in different ways, the main reason being to 'sustain couplehood' as long as possible. The couple perform 'dignity work' (Örulv & Nikku 2007; see also Öhlander, this volume, Chapter 4), or in other words they 'walk a tight-rope'. Both partners balance their actions in everyday life. The people with dementia actively avoid situations that could have an effect on their dignity of identity, and their cognitively intact spouses try to maintain the involvement of their ill partner in order not to humiliate them, and stress their former achievements.

Nordenfelt (this volume, Chapter 2) argues that the dignity of wisdom can be applied to older people as a group. But can we consider people with dementia wise? They have lived a long time and of course have knowledge of life, but if you forget large parts of your life and achievements, are you still wise? The challenge for dementia care is to see that the person with dementia has knowledge about life and to listen to their life story, even if the story is mixed up in time, and most achievement and efforts are in the past. And we should bear in mind that for the person with dementia the achievements in the past may be relived in the present. But how do we listen to their wisdom when their voices have faded away? Here there are no simple answers. In most spousal relation-ships the life story is often shared with a partner, but because of memory problems their common life story becomes shattered, and the spouse therefore has difficulty in 'reshaping the boat' alone.

Acknowledgements

The longitudinal study was conducted in collaboration with Ulla Lundh, associate professor at Linköping University, Sweden, and with Mike Nolan, professor at the Sheffield Institute for Studies on Ageing, University of Sheffield, United Kingdom. The interviews with the spouses were conducted by Ulla Lundh. The interviews with the people with dementia and the nursing assistants were conducted by Ingrid Hellström.

References

Bamford, C. & Bruce, E. (2000) Defining the outcomes of community care: the perspective of older people with dementia and their carers. *Ageing and Society*, **20**, 543–570.

Bond, J. & Corner, L. (2001) Researching dementia: are there unique methodological chal-lenges for health services research? *Ageing and Society*, **21**, 95–116.

Corbin, J.M. & Strauss, A. (1988) *Unending Work and Care: Managing Chronic Illness at Home.* Jossey Bass, San Francisco, CA.

Cotrell, V. & Schultz, R. (1993) The perspective of the patient with Alzheimer's disease: A neglected dimension of dementia research. *Gerontologist*, **33**, 205–211.

Crisp, J. (1999) Towards a partnership in maintaining personhood. In: *Dementia Care: Developing Partnerships in Practice* (eds T. Adams and C.L. Clarke), pp. 92–120. Baillière Tindall, London.

Dewing, J. (2002) From ritual to relationship: a person-centred approach to consent in qualitative research with older people who have dementia. *Dementia*, **1**, 157–171.

Forbat, L. (2003) Relationships difficulties in dementia care: a discursive analysis of two women's accounts. *Dementia*, **2**, 76–84.

Goldsmith, M. (1996) *Hearing the Voice of People with Dementia: Opportunities and Obstacles*. Jessica Kingsley, London.

Hellström, I. (2005) Exploring 'Couplehood' in Dementia: a Constructivist Grounded Theory Study. PhD thesis, Linköping University.

Hellström, I., Nolan, M. & Lundh, U. (2007) Sustaining 'couplehood'. Spouses' strategies for living positively with dementia. *Dementia*, **6**, 383–409.

Hirschfield, M.J. (1983) Home care versus institutionalisation: family caregiving and senile brain disease. *International Journal of Nursing Studies*, **20**, 23–32.

Holm, S. (2001) Autonomy, authenticity, or best interest: everyday decision-making and persons with dementia. *Medicine Health Care and Philosophy*, **4**, 153–159.

Kaplan, L. (2001) A couplehood typology for spouses of institutionalised persons with Alzheimer's disease: perceptions of 'we'–'I', *Family Relations*, **50**, 87–98.

Keady, J. (1999) The Dynamics of Dementia: a Modified Grounded Theory Study. PhD thesis, University of Wales, Bangor.

Kirk, H. (1995) Da alderen blev en diagnose [When old age became a diagnosis]. PhD thesis, Munksgaard, Copenhagen.

Kitwood, T. (1997a) *Dementia Reconsidered: the Person Comes First*. Open University Press, Buckingham.

Kitwood, T. (1997b) The concept of personhood and its relevance for a new culture of dementia care. In: *Caregiving in Dementia: Research and Applications*, Vol. **2** (eds B.M.L. Miesen and G.M.M. Jones), pp. 3–13. Routledge, London.

Kitwood, T. & Bredin, K. (1992) Towards a theory of dementia care: personhood and well-being. *Ageing and Society*, **12**, 269–287.

Montgomery, R.J.V. & Williams, K.N. (2001) Implications of differential impacts of care-giving for future research on Alzheimer care. *Aging and Mental Health*, **5** (Suppl. 1), 23–34.

Motenko, A.K. (1989) The frustrations, gratifications and well-being of dementia caregivers. *Gerontologist*, **29**, 166–172.

Nolan, M.R., Grant, G. & Keady, J. (1996) *Understanding Family Care: a Multidimensional Model of Caring and Coping*. Open University Press, Buckingham.

Nolan, M., Ryan, T., Enderby, P. & Reid, D. (2002) Towards a more inclusive vision of dementia care practice and research. *Dementia*, **1**, 193–211.

O'Connor, D., Phinney, A., Small, J. et al. (2007) Personhood in dementia care. Developing a research agenda for broadening the vision. *Dementia*, **6**, 121–142.

Örulv, L. & Nikku, N. (2007) Dignity work in dementia care. Sketching a microethical analysis. *Dementia*, **6**, 507–525.

Page, S. & Fletcher, T. (2006) Auguste D. one hundred years on: 'the person' not 'the case'. *Dementia*, **5**, 571–583.

Perry, J. (1995) A Study of Women Caregiving to Husbands Who Have Alzheimer's Disease: Family Know-How as a Process of Interpretive Caring. PhD thesis, University of Washington, Washington DC.

Phinney, A. (2002) Living with the symptoms of Alzheimer's disease. In: *The Person with Alzheimer's Disease* (eds P. Braudy Harris), pp. 49–74. Johns Hopkins University Press, Baltimore, MD.

Post, S. (1995) *The Moral Challenge of Alzheimer's disease*. Johns Hopkins University Press, Baltimore, MD.

Sabat, S. (2001) *The Experience of Alzheimer's Disease: Life Through a Tangled Veil*. Blackwell, Oxford.

Sabat, S. (2002) Surviving manifestations of selfhood in Alzheimer's disease. A case study. *Dementia*, **1**, 25–36.

Sällström, C. (1994) Spouses' Experiences of Living with a Partner with Alzheimer's Disease. PhD thesis, University of Umeå.

Schulz, R. & Williamson, G.M. (1997) The measurement of caregiver outcomes in AD research. *Alzheimer's Disease and Related Disorders*, **11**, (Suppl. 6), 1–6.

Swane, C.E. (1996) Hverdagen med demens [Everyday life with dementia]. PhD thesis, Munksgaard, Copenhagen.

Whitlach, C.J. (2001) Including the person with dementia in family care-giving research. *Aging and Mental Health*, **5**, (Suppl. 1) 20–22.

Wilkinson, H. (2002) Including people with dementia in research: methods and motivations. In: *The Perspectives of People with Dementia: Research Methods and Motivations* (ed. H. Wilkinson), pp. 9–24. Jessica Kingsley, London.

Woods, R.T. (2001) Discovering the person with Alzheimer's disease: cognitive, emotional and behavioural aspects. *Aging and Mental Health*, **5**, (Suppl. 1), 7–16.

6. *Caring for Older People: Why Dignity Matters – the European Experience*

Win Tadd and Michael Calnan

Introduction

Although many older people in Europe now enjoy better health and greater affluence than ever before, a pessimistic image of increasing age and the attendant discrimination against older people remains widespread (HAS 2000 1998; Levenson 2002; Ray et al. 2006). The challenges posed by an ageing population include a shrinking workforce, pressure on pensions and public funds, increasing demand for health and social care, social diversity, social exclusion and gender issues. These challenges, which affect all European countries to a greater or lesser degree, cannot be met if older people remain the subject of negative stereotyping and discriminatory practices, which detract from their social worth and self-esteem.

The right to, and the need for, dignity is frequently cited in European policy documents relating to the health and social care of older people (DH 2000, 2001a, 2001b, 2006a; MHSA 1997; Brazinová et al. 2004). In the UK, the NHS Plan (DH 2000) uses the term on a number of occasions (Chapter 15 is entitled 'Dignity, security, and independence in old age') and the National Service Framework for Older People explicitly mentions dignity in relation to person-centred care (DH 2001a). More recently, the UK National Director for Older People presented the next steps for the National Service Framework in a report entitled *A New Ambition for Old Age* (DH 2006a). The report describes how some staff demonstrate deep-rooted negative attitudes and behaviours towards older people and it concludes that much more will have to be done if all older people are to receive care that is humane and dignified. As a first step, both the English and Welsh Departments of Health (DH 2006b; WAG 2007), have established Dignity in Care initiatives to ensure that all older people are treated with dignity when using health and social care services. In Wales, a Commissioner for Older People took up her appointment in April 2008 and is responsible for ensuring that the rights of older people in Wales are upheld. This is the first post of its kind in Europe. These initiatives are intended to create zero tolerance towards violations of dignity in any care setting and will focus on inspection and regulation, complaint management and the education and training of all health and social work professionals.

119

A similar emphasis is placed on dignity in other European countries. For example, the government of the Slovak Republic has adopted a *Charter of Patients' Rights* (Brazinová et al. 2004) which states that the 'rights of patients are based on the right to human dignity, self-determination and autonomy' and in Sweden the 1997 Health Act states that 'Care shall be given with respect for the equal value of all human beings and for the dignity of the individual' (MHSA 1997).

The importance of promoting dignity is also emphasised in professional codes and international declarations of human rights (UNO 1948; Council of Europe 1997; ICN 2000; NMC 2004). Yet concerns about the standards of care for older people abound (Tadd & Bayer 2001; Baggott et al. 2005). Although many of today's older people are more able to pursue their interests than their predecessors, through better education and improved financial and physical well-being, the last years of life are still characterised by hardships such as poverty, chronic illness, disability, dementia, increased dependence and social isolation (Calnan et al. 2003). A major issue for many European societies is therefore how to ensure that older people can live out their days with dignity.

Why dignity? There is evidence that positive health and social outcomes result when people feel more valued and respected; are involved in care decisions; maintain a positive self-regard; and are able to exercise direction over their lives (Kenny 1990; Bensink et al. 1992; Brillhart & Johnson 1997; Ranzijn et al. 1998; Tadd et al. 2002; Walsh & Kowanko 2002; Beach et al. 2005; Glendinning et al. 2006). Furthermore, once dignity is marginalised, there is a danger that neglect and disregard will become the norm and that staff morale will plummet, as staff members themselves are 'brutalised' by 'uncaring' systems (HAS 2000 1998; DH 2001b; Tadd & Bayer 2001; Baggott et al. 2005). Such consequences have been routinely uncovered in investigations into patient abuse (CHI 2003). All this suggests that the perception of patients as people possessing dignity is of the utmost importance in practice, and considerations of dignity should be a central element in the provision of high-quality care.

Dignity is, however, a complex concept and difficult to define. Without clarification of the concept, any aspiration to recognise, respect and promote the dignity of individuals is not only subject to wide interpretation but also in danger of degenerating into mere slogans (van Hooft et al. 1995). It is therefore surprising that relatively little research has been undertaken into the meaning of dignity, especially with reference to the most vulnerable groups. Some analysis of the concept and its importance for nursing has been undertaken (Pokorny 1989; Haddock 1996; Söderberg et al. 1997; Gallagher & Seedhouse 2002; Jacelon 2004), but systematic evidence as to how those providing care for older people see dignity, or how they promote dignified care, is limited (Seedhouse & Gallagher 2002; Woolhead et al. 2003).

The study reported here involved eliciting the meaning that older people ascribed to dignity and discovering their experiences of dignity and dignified treatment and care. It also explored how health and social care professionals viewed dignity and its importance or otherwise in the care of older people, together with what young and middle-aged adults thought about dignity, old age and older people's lives. In this chapter we describe the results of this 3-year comparative study undertaken in six European countries before drawing conclusions.

6.1 The Dignity and Older Europeans study

The Dignity and Older Europeans (DOE) project was funded b
mission and involved a partnership of nurses, philosophers, sociolog
clinicians, health service researchers and NGOs. Very briefly, it involv
The first was a review and analysis of the literature, development of a thee
of dignity and creation of a large bibliographic database. The empirical phase
of qualitative analysis of data from 265 focus groups involving 1320 participa
the UK, Spain, France, Sweden, Slovakia and Ireland. The third phase involve
development of inter-professional educational materials and policy and servi
recommendations.

Although a full account of the study is beyond the remit of this chapter, detailed
versions of the methodology can be found in Calnan & Tadd (2005); of the philosophical
model in Nordenfelt (2003, 2004) and Nordenfelt & Edgar (2005); and of the European
findings as a whole in Bayer et al. (2005), Arino-Blasco et al. (2005) and Stratton & Tadd
(2005).

6.1.1   The model of human dignity

The meaning and importance of the concept of dignity is frequently contested (Macklin
2003), and much of the contention concerns the congruence between its subjective
interpretation and objective implementation (Edgar 2004; Nordenfelt 2004). Spiegelberg
(1970) discussed the vagueness and inconsistencies of the term 'dignity' and distinguished between 'dignity in general' and 'human dignity' in particular. Dignity in
general is subjective, often a matter of degree, and can be gained or lost, while human
dignity 'refers to the minimum dignity which belongs to every human being as a human
being. There are no degrees, it is equal for everyone and cannot be gained or lost' (p.
42). The model developed in this study, and discussed in Chapter 2, describes four types
of dignity, three of which reflect Spiegelberg's 'dignity in general' (dignity of merit,
dignity of moral stature and dignity of identity), while the fourth equates to 'human
dignity' (*Menschenwürde*).

To briefly summarise this model for the purposes of this chapter:

Dignity of merit
Dignity of merit concerns social worth and is often applied to the status of certain offices
or occupations, such as that of cabinet minister, bishop, doctor or even aristocrat or
monarch. These are *formal dignities of merit* related to notions of rights and the inherent
respect attached to such positions. Informal dignities of merit exist when people are
recognised for their achievements and thus gain public respect. Examples include artis-
tic, scientific or athletic prowess.

Dignity of moral stature
This type of dignity emphasises the importance of a person's moral integrity and is
often reflected in their behaviour. If people are able to live according to their moral
principles, they will experience a sense of dignity. By contrast, someone who behaves
in a cowardly way, who is cruel to another individual, or who for whatever reason acts
contrary to their moral principles, may not only lose self-respect but also the

rees, as one's moral standards may be

gnity of identity is related to self-respect
on. It can be violated by physical inter-
such as humiliation or embarrassment.
self, physical identity and the ability to
A cruel person might violate another's
their private sphere, physically hurting
g them from social interaction. Any of
of self-worth and therefore their dignity.
arelessness such as exposing their bodies
the person's perception of their identity
eir sense of themselves as an autonomous
and responsible person is challeng seem to resemble a passive object, subject
to the whims of others.

The dignity of identity also refers to the ability to construct a meaningful account of one's life, with the dignified person being able to provide a positive description, either as an individual or as a member of a group. When dignity of identity exists, individuals have a sense of completeness enabling them to share positive relationships with others and a sense of inclusion in their community. As such they are able to make sense of their lives. When cultural resources to recount a positive narrative are lacking, feelings of exclusion may result.

Human dignity

The final type of dignity identified within the model is human dignity (*Menschenwürde*), which implies a moral requirement to respect all human beings, regardless of their social, mental or physical properties (UNO 1948). Human dignity, in Spiegelberg's (1970) terminology, acknowledges that dignity is not simply a matter of what human beings feel or what is recognised by the moral culture of a particular society, but is grounded in what it is to be human. At its core is the concept of 'humanness', something that cannot be taken away or lost. Human capacities recognised as deserving dignity include consciousness, the ability to reason, the capacity for self-reflection, the facility to determine one's way of life and select one's norms and values. These abilities are commonly referred to as the capacity for autonomy. The right to respect for autonomy and the moral obligation of 'respect for persons', therefore, are seen to flow from human dignity, while experiencing the dignities of merit, moral stature and identity might be described as preconditions for a sense of self-respect.

6.1.2 Methodology

Our main concern was to explore the meanings, beliefs and values regarding dignity of different groups of people from their own perspectives, and focus groups were chosen as an appropriate method of data collection (Kitzinger 2000). The strengths and weaknesses of focus groups as a qualitative methodology have been well documented (Kidd & Parshall 2000; Bloor et al. 2000; Webb & Kevern 2001). They are particularly appropriate in cross-cultural studies, as they can elicit cultural values and examine how linguistic exchanges operate within a given cultural context (Kitzinger & Barbour 1999).

Sampling

Participants were purposely targeted and selected to maximise the variation in socio-economic status, ethnicity, gender, place of abode, family circumstances, age, level of fitness/frailty and membership of clubs and groups (Table 6.1). Also, the homogeneity of several of the individual focus group sessions was promoted, partly to encourage open discussion (for example, separate sessions with young, middle-aged, and 'young-old' and 'old-old' adults were held) and in some cases to avoid potential distractions as with mixing different categories and grades of health and social-care professionals. Although it is generally recommended that 8–10 participants is the optimum size for a focus group (Kitzinger 1995), after conducting several groups, it was evident that groups with more than 7 participants lacked cohesion and that the optimum was 4–7. Each group had a moderator and assistant. The discussions were audio-taped and transcribed verbatim. Before any data collection, ethical approval from appropriate bodies was obtained.

We held 265 focus group sessions, and 2 individual interviews were held with the 3 groups of participants. More specifically, 391 older people took part in 91 focus groups and 2 individual interviews. The sessions were held in various settings including hospitals, exercise and leisure classes, sheltered housing schemes, community health facilities and councils, nursing homes, various senior clubs, the University of the Third Age forum, private and community residential facilities, community centres, day hospitals, and general medical practices spread across urban and rural areas. The majority (283) of the older participants were women, and participant ages ranged from 50 to 95 (241 were aged under 79 and 115 were over 80 years of age). The majority lived at home (see Table 6.1), and participants with and without disability were included. Undertaking focus group sessions at different sites and in different contexts increased the likelihood of identifying diverse discourses as well as enhancing reliability and validity (Kidd & Parshall 2000).

In addition, 85 focus group sessions were held in various locations with 424 health-care and social-care workers, professionals and managers. The participants were purposely selected to reflect different occupations, levels of seniority, percentages of time spent with older people, and clinical and organisational settings. Among the participants were nurses, geriatricians, care assistants, social workers, physiotherapists and their assistants, home-care managers, medical, nursing and social work students, occupational therapists, speech therapists, psychologists, service managers, teachers and social workers. Their work settings included long-stay and continuing care facilities, acute hospitals, community hospitals, domiciliary care, and private residential or nursing homes (see Table 6.1). On average, 79% of the participants' working hours were dedicated to older people. The majority were women (369), and the mean age was 41 years.

There were 89 focus groups with 505 younger (296) and middle-aged (209) adults. Again, specific recruitment ensured a wide mix of participants in relation to age, gender, marital status, educational attainment, occupation, place of abode and experience of caring for older people. The 296 younger adults were aged from 13 to 30 years, and the

Table 6.1 Characteristics of the focus group participants

Older people		Young adults		Middle-aged adults		Professionals	
Age (years)		**Age (years)**		**Age (years)**		**Age (years)**	
Mean	76	Mean	20.5	Mean	48.75	Average	41
Range	50–95	Range	13–30	Range	31–81	Range	18–77
Marital status		Marital status		Marital status		**Occupation**	
Widowed	190	Widowed	0	Widowed	6	Care assistant	111
Married	114	Married	30	Married	146	Physiotherapy assistant	8
Unmarried	31	Unmarried	261	Never married	28	Physiotherapists	14
Separated/divorced	25	Separated/divorced	1	Separated/divorced	23	Occupational therapist	10
Missing data	31	Missing data	4	Missing data	6	Social worker	24
Educational level		Educational level		Educational level		Managers	40
Basic[a]	111	Basic[a]	1	Basic[1]	16	Physician	42
Secondary[b]	127	Secondary[b]	205	Secondary[2]	54	Medical student	4
Tertiary	88	Tertiary	89	Tertiary	133	Nursing student	2
Missing data[c]	65	Missing data	1	Missing data	5	Social work student	8
						Other[d]	26
Location of current home		**Location of current home**		**Location of current home**		**Location of work**	
City	164	City	207	City	104	Domiciliary	42
Town	60	Town	62	Town	61	Community	122
Rural	9	Rural	26	Rural	43	Hospitals	163
Missing data	158	Missing data	1	Missing data	0	Residential care	119
						Other	4
						Unemployed	1
						Missing data	15

Previous occupation	
Manual	166
Non-manual	134
Missing data	91
Living arrangement	
Lives alone	101
Lives with spouse	97
Lives with relatives	23
Residential homes	7
Residential care	54
Missing data	114
Female	**283**
Male	**108**
Total	**391**

Occupation	
Manual	9
Routine and semi-routine	4
Intermediate	14
Managerial/professional	44
Students	220
Unemployed or never worked	3
Missing data	91
Experience of care of older people	
None	187
Previous	69
Current	33
Missing data	7
Female	**196**
Male	**100**
Total	**296**

Occupation	
Manual	15
Routine and semi-routine	26
Intermediate	35
Managerial/professional	109
Students	0
Unemployed or never worked	19
Missing data	4
Experience of care of older people	
None	92
Previous	65
Current	46
Missing data	5
Female	**131**
Male	**78**
Total	**209**

Percentage of time spent with older people	
Mean	79
Range	0–100
Female	**369**
Male	**55**
Total	**424**

Notes: [a] Left school without any qualifications. [b] Gained national school leaving certificates. [c] Data not collected in Sweden due to variations in educational system [d] Includes dieticians, pharmacists, psychologists, domestic staff and ward clerks.

209 middle-aged adults from 31 to 65 years (see Table 6.1). Once again women were predominant in both groups, but particularly in the middle-aged group. The middle-aged participants reported more direct experience of caring for older people than the younger adults.

The character of a focus group discussion is somewhere between the discourse of meetings and conversations (Kidd & Parshall 2000). The facilitators encouraged spontaneous rather than 'meeting-like' discourse. While the interview guides had broad, open questions, groups usually began with general and spontaneous discussion before focusing on issues directly related to the meaning of dignity and its experience in daily life and health and social care. When 'dignity' emerged spontaneously in the discussions the exchanges were guided by specific questions; when it did not, it was directly prompted, often facilitated by visual images (Calnan & Tadd 2005).

Analysis
Data collection and inductive thematic analysis continued concurrently according to the method of constant comparison (Strauss & Corbin 1998) until no new information was forthcoming, thus theoretical saturation was achieved. All discussions were audio-taped and fully transcribed. Analysis was a two-stage process and involved detailed scrutiny of the verbatim transcripts to identify and open-code segments of discourse or ideas; thereafter coding was undertaken to arrange the codes into themes (the computer software package Atlas Ti 4.1 was used). Initially, in each country two researchers independently coded the transcribed data, before comparing codes and reaching agreement by discussion when necessary. Negative or deviant cases (examples that contradicted emerging themes) were investigated closely. A second analysis of the data was then undertaken in a similar manner using the four types of dignity identified in the model as an organising thematic framework. The aim was to explore the consistency between the participants' accounts of dignity and the model, and it is this analysis that is presented in this chapter. There was considerable consistency between the model of dignity and the participants' views.

6.2   Findings

6.2.1   Dignity of merit
Participants' discussions reflected this type of dignity in various ways, and although generally it was not much discussed by either older participants or young and middle-aged adults, some relevant points were made. For example, older participants emphasised that an individual's status and sense of self-worth are frequently provided by their employment, which provides them with an income and guarantees their place as consumers. Retirement, especially when enforced, threatened the sense of self-worth, by undermining older people's merit as 'contributors' and reducing their disposable income. The threat of poverty due to inadequate pension provision was mentioned in all countries and older people saw this as evidence of their lack of social value within contemporary societies:

... because part of dignity does relate to money. Unfortunately in my view we need to get adequate pensions so we are equal in society and don't need concessions (72-year-old man, UK).

Many middle-aged participants also reflected on older people's lack of financial resources, highlighting its impact on social exclusion and the increased sense of isolation experienced by many older people:

That again boils down to finance. The majority of the older population are on a state pension and that goes absolutely nowhere. That doesn't give people dignity, it is literally just keeping them on or even below the poverty line. They can't afford to enjoy themselves, they can barely keep themselves (50-year-old man, UK).

Young adults generally concurred with this view but they also believed that older people deserved special esteem for the contributions they had made to society during their lives. These participants frequently expressed the view that older people deserved respect for their dignity of merit due to the wisdom they had acquired from long lives and varied experiences:

On a positive side it's the experience, theoretically, a kind of wisdom ... Learning through time. This is what touches me particularly (30-year-old man, France).

I mentioned the word respect earlier, and I wasn't just thinking of the physical respect of helping somebody across the road, or standing back, or giving them a seat, that kind of thing, but also respect for their opinions and accumulated wisdom. We are told that in some primitive societies the elders are the most respected. In some cases, that is possibly true of our own society, but I think largely only if they have already made a name for themselves, or in the family, or in society, but I am inclined to think that generally the older person's opinions are, or can be, discounted, as the youngsters say 'old hat' (56-year-old woman, Ireland).

Professional participants discussed the unequal access to services experienced by older people as an infringement of their dignity of merit as it reflected the lack of social worth afforded to older people:

It is like, they are old, they cannot manage any more. And they could be really sick but they are just given this label. They are seen almost as a nuisance. If there is a general medical team on call they may be giving out about how everyone we get in is elderly as if they were less entitled to medical care than if they were younger (female geriatrician, Ireland).

I was visited by a doctor, an employee of the health insurance company, who asked me why I prescribed drugs for older people and did not think of young patients who would miss out on appropriate treatment because of the older people (female psychiatrist, Slovakia).

Professionals' comments reflected the direct experiences of older people themselves:

Society seems to want you to become helpless. If you need a knee or a hip replacement that would improve your quality of life and make you a younger older person if you like, but you are at the bottom of that list … surgery that would improve the quality of life, make you more independent … to me that would be saving money, but they just leave people to get worse and worse (64-year-old woman, UK).

Every time I went to him with a minor complaint he would say, 'Sure, aren't you very well considering what age you are'. That was all the sympathy I got! (70-year-old woman, Ireland).

The dignity of merit was also a crucially important issue for professionals themselves. They recognised that their colleagues, members of the public and the media often saw caring for older people as unglamorous and of low status. Acute care and high-tech specialisms were viewed as more desirable sectors in which to work and thus people choosing to work with older people, whether in hospital or in social or community care, were often seen as unworthy or incapable of working in other areas, and the term 'Cinderella service' was frequently used to describe such work. Such attitudes impacted adversely on the professionals' dignity of merit, and professional participants claimed that the low status afforded to care of older people had resulted in inadequate financial and human resources and impoverished care environments.

And you have to have the right environment for treating people with dignity, some of our real estate is very poor … It would be easy to maintain dignity if all patients were in single rooms so you didn't have to worry about the fact that the curtains always seem to be inadequate and all the nice curtains have disappeared to the laundry never to be seen again (male geriatrician, UK).

For professionals in particular, the dignity of merit was closely related to the second type of dignity, that of moral stature.

6.2.2   Dignity of moral stature
Discussions within the professional focus groups reflected this variety of dignity, with many emphasising how morally destructive caring for older people can be as a result of continually working within poorly resourced systems. This meant that the 'patient as a person' was often forgotten and emphasis was placed on getting the job done. This left professionals with little job satisfaction or self-esteem.

If only you didn't have to struggle all the time to get things, access things for patients, access equipment, access tests, the whole journey would be a better experience for patients. … when people operate under huge pressure it's very easy to depersonalise the people that you are dealing with (female geriatrician, UK).

Lack of time meant that not only was the dignity of patients and service users violated, but also that of the professionals. Job satisfaction and pride in one's work were difficult to realise in such situations, while providing levels of care below the standards required by the respective professions severely dented the professionals' dignity of moral stature. Many stated that they worked hard to adhere to their professional ethics and altruistic values as these helped them treat people with dignity and promoted their own dignity of moral stature. Thus it was in the context of barriers to the provision of dignified care that professionals' comments reflected this type of dignity.

And we already talked about this, it affects our dignity, I think this is where it touches us – in our dignity as professionals (qualified nurse, France)

It [care of older people] is so badly perceived, as if the institution is bad, so those working in the place are bad (nursing aide, France).

I have worked with 28 people, and had lots of work, but you did it with all your loving care …, and leaving there with your head high, it fulfils you [sic]. Then, working in geriatrics and also having 28 patients and leaving with the feeling that you were better the faster you did the work, but how you did it didn't matter. And feeling like you worked in a factory, that the more output you produced, the more you were appreciated (female care assistant, Spain).

Within these discussions, a loop effect was evident, wherein a low-valued care sector generated a lack of respect for professionals and older people alike. This, together with underfunding, resulted in impoverished environments, a high turnover and lack of suitable personnel, which in turn resulted in increasing workloads. The old aphorism – that older people are second-class citizens who get second-class services from those perceived to be second-class professionals – still seemed pertinent to many professionals.

For older participants this type of dignity was also important and it was discussed in relation to many aspects of their lives. At a personal level they described how the older person's own behaviour could impact on their self-respect and therefore their dignity of moral stature. Acting with decorum, especially in unpleasant or offensive circumstances, was seen as an indicator of dignity:

I don't know, I think as far as one can be dignified it's the way one responds to adversity or disrespect for others, insults from others, mocking ridicule from others. It's a measure of your dignity, how well you respond. … Are you conducting yourself well? I think that's dignity (male older adult, UK).

To feel dignified you have to live right (67-year-old man, Spain).

Others mentioned the need to keep one's temper and have good manners if one was to maintain dignity. Such comments are interesting, in that not only do they provide insight into older people's views of what it means to behave in a dignified manner, but they may provide an explanation as to why older people are often described as passive, uncomplaining recipients of care, regardless of the standard of that care (Walker 1999; Gilleard & Higgs 2000). Making a fuss, complaining or indeed reacting angrily to poor care would detract from the individual's perception of themselves as a moral person.

Acceptance of the fact that one was becoming old and accepting the inevitable changes rather than pursuing youth was claimed by some to reflect the dignity of moral stature – a view which was also held by other participants:

No, I don't think it [dressing in a way that does not suit one's age] *gives dignity, you just have to look at the old women who want to play at being girls. That would not have happened years ago* (83-year-old woman, France).

I think it's also behaving, you know in a respectful manner. Dressing in a manner appropriate to your age.

I don't think I agree with that. People should be able to dress for themselves not for others.

Well, I don't think it's very dignified to be the age of 65 and wear a miniskirt for instance (53- and 55-year-old women, UK).

Younger and middle-aged adults also discussed self-respect as an important factor in having and maintaining one's dignity. Self-respect, however, is not exclusively related to the dignity of moral stature but was claimed by many participants to impact on the dignity of identity as it affected one's perception of oneself.

6.2.3 Dignity of identity

It was this type of dignity that was reflected most in older people's discussions of dignity or rather 'indignity'. Illness, disability, poverty or old age can threaten the dignity of identity. When older people become infirm and frail, their disabilities and illnesses are often irreversible and therefore their identity may be severely altered. Challenges to dignity may also occur when individuals can no longer care for themselves or move independently, as they risk intrusion in the most private spheres of their lives.

All participants highlighted the impact of ageist stereotypes on this type of dignity. Negative images of older people in advertising and the mass media reinforced feelings of marginalisation and inhibited acknowledgement of older people's diversity, their potential and competences. The key themes drawn from the participants' accounts that impact on this type of dignity are identified below.

Being a burden

Particularly relevant was the fear of becoming a burden, as many older people believed that this was how society saw them. Media headlines emphasising the cost of older people's care, ageist or negative images on birthday cards, in popular entertainment or on road signs, were all cited as evidence of these claims. Feeling or perceiving oneself to be a burden also denied older people the opportunity to provide a positive description of their lives:

The dignity of a human being lasts while you serve yourself. When you can't serve yourself, you've lost it. You need everything from everyone else. And then you're not living any more, because you see that people have no choice but to do it (67-year- old male, Spain).

You're a burden on society and you're ostracised. That's a complete lack of dignity in my view ... they're regarded by the rest of the community ... as being a burden ... you should be a part of society and regarded as such (88-year-old man, UK).

The old are a burden. They smile at the old people but this smile is cold, only to fulfil duty, it is without love and feeling (83-year-old woman, Slovakia).

Professionals confirmed that many older people expressed negative views of how they are viewed in society, particularly as burdens to both their families and the state. Some professionals also claimed that just by needing care, one's dignity of identity and sense of self could be diminished:

> *A requirement for care results in a lack of dignity ... We are dignified if we handle everything ourselves and we don't cause anyone any trouble ... And then, of course, comes old age ... few people reach old age without having to ask for some sort of help. That can really impact negatively on how they see themselves* (male geriatrician, UK).

From many of the participants' comments it appeared that perceptions about the need for care, especially on an ongoing basis, have acquired evaluative connotations, which reflect on both the recipient and the caregiver. The idea that increasing old age (which many of us are now able to look forward to) may also result in the need for care appears to threaten the experience of dignity. Potential recipients of care feared being a burden and expressed shame at being in need of assistance or being dependent, so that not requiring care seems to have become a measure of individual dignity. This view of care in Western communities was described by Keith et al. (1990) in a study comparing American and Chinese communities. Older Americans were, like their European counterparts, concerned that they should not become dependent, whereas the Chinese elders hoped they had raised children who would take care of them if or when they did (p. 260).

Respect and self-respect
Younger participants, in particular, commented upon both the self and other-regarding aspects of 'respect' and how this may impinge upon the experience of dignity of identity. For example, the participant below describes how our view of ourselves and thus our self-respect are shaped by others' responses to us, emphasising the importance of being shown respect:

> *I think there are two elements to it. There is how I think your personhood is perceived by others and I think with dignity you tend to associate an element of respect given to you ... there's also the level of personal dignity, you know, where how you feel about yourself and how you feel that you can fulfil certain roles, and I think being shown respect greatly impacts on our self-respect, so for me it's [dignity] a mixture of both of them* (28-year-old man, UK).

Older participants emphasised how there was little respect shown to older people in today's society, not only through the widespread negative images mentioned above, but also at the level of individual behaviour, and they cited how derogatory slang terms such as 'cotton buds' or 'wrinklies' were used to address them This, they claimed, demonstrated how they were seen as figures of fun, which greatly affected their sense of identity and therefore their dignity.

Invisibility
Participants also referred to the impact of the ageing process on the dignity of identity. Older adults in particular mentioned the anonymity and invisibility which getting older brought:

131

You get quite anonymous, I think, you get grey hair and become anonymous. I don't know, but if there are a lot of young people, they tend to overlook you, they chat amongst themselves and they don't address you unless they want something.

M: *Do other people agree?*

Yes, I think young people are in their little clique and even within the family you find that they will talk amongst themselves, and you think: Well, am I here as well? (75- and 84-year-old women, UK).

Older participants also described many instances of being made to feel invisible, as though they did not count or had ceased to exist.

I'm thinking of a patient who had difficulty in walking and was in a wheelchair. When we went down to the city to buy her new clothes the shop assistant addressed me, over her head! (67-year-old woman, Sweden).

Personal appearance
Older participants also believed that it was essential to look presentable and respectable in order to promote and maintain their dignity, regardless of age, illness, disability or income.

I think even though I am in a wheelchair, I like to think I look good and that makes me feel good. They say 'Doesn't she look nice, she has got her lipstick on'; and yes, I like it when they say I look nice and it makes you feel good. The same when you go and have your hair done, it makes you feel good too (74-year-old woman, UK).

It's a dignified position because their appearance is good (80-year-old woman, Spain)

They look like dignified, noble people (77-year-old woman, Spain)

It's also the way they dress, and groom. When you see that the person is clean, that it's a person who has been treated with dignity. And they live in a normal healthy environment (75-year-old woman, Spain).

The attention that health and social care staff paid to older people's appearance was seen as a measure of respect and a way of promoting dignity.

They treated her with respect and she looked it, always beautifully dressed (75-year-old man, Ireland).

Despite recognising the importance of personal appearance in promoting and maintaining an older person's dignity, many professional participants admitted that they often forgot such aspects of personal care, which could result in those they cared for feeling undignified:

It's the same with things like their hair, you know, making sure their hair is tidy and making sure they have got their glasses, teeth in, all these things are important for dignity (female staff nurse, UK).

Or if they wear make-up, then they have their make-up on, and like the hairdresser being here today (female staff nurse, UK).

You have got to remember though, because sometimes you forget about their teeth because they are inside the mouth and you can't see them (female student nurse, UK).

I rarely forget teeth but I always forget hair (female health-care assistant, UK).

Other professionals commented on how institutional living can rob individuals of their identity:

At a nursing home, often the person admitted gets cancelled out ... . People seem to stop being themselves. There are nursing homes where everyone has to wear a gown. Please, tell me what for! People want to dress as they like or do their own thing, don't they? (female social worker, Spain).

Middle-aged adults, rather than their younger counterparts, also believed that personal appearance was an important aspect of maintaining older people's dignity. In particular it mattered when others were responsible for assisting older people in their self-presentation. A number of these participants spoke at length about the impact that entry to residential care had and how such personal aspects were frequently neglected. One woman spoke about being asked to bring jogging trousers for her father to wear to avoid incontinence. Throughout his life her father had always dressed formally and she felt that to make him dress any differently would be to remove an important part of his identity and thus assault his dignity.

Communication

For many older participants, the greatest assaults on the dignity of identity resulted from contact with health or social services. Communication practices were particularly highlighted as one of the areas where older people's dignity of identity was infringed. Examples included being ignored or being treated as an 'object':

I went into this particular specialist and he had an assistant. Instead of talking to me he was writing all the time, I could have been an elephant. He said, 'take her in there and tell her to strip down' and I just said, 'Am I invisible?' (66-year-old woman, Ireland).

You know exactly what to do, you change the nappy and wash the old person. And it's just a matter of routine, you do it and you actually forget that it's a person lying there (female nursing assistant, Sweden).

To be ignored or treated as an object, to be manipulated, is perhaps the most straightforward example of a humiliating act. The person's capacity to understand and their right to make autonomous decisions are both infringed. At best, the person is reduced to the dependent state of a child and at worst it is one of the most drastic forms of social exclusion.

Another problem was the way in which older people were addressed. Older people decried the use of pet names or first names on a routine basis, as this reflected their position of unequal power and reduced them to feelings of child-like dependency:

That sense of inferiority can be subtly reinforced by first naming, since to some people it conjures up memories of helplessness in the classroom. Choice hardly exists … You are Tom or Mary before you know where you are (older woman, UK).

… if she had been addressed 'Your Ladyship' during all her life, and she was about 90, why couldn't she have been allowed this during her last two weeks (86-year-old woman, Sweden).

Professionals also recognised the importance of not patronising older people by speaking to them as though they were children, such as using first or pet names:

I think in some situations you can turn older people into children by the way you treat them by using their first name or by using endearments such as 'dear', 'duck' and 'love'. It reduces them to how you would treat a child … (specialist nurse, UK).

Humiliation, ridicule and embarrassment
Many older people reported feelings of humiliation, embarrassment or being ridiculed in their dealings with health and social care professionals, all of which impacted on their dignity of identity as it left them unable to give a positive account of their lives. Being ridiculed in particular was also another means of reducing older people and making them feel childish:

There is another kind of not respecting dignity, that isn't as severe, it is in little details … Like laughing at someone when they've said the wrong word, because when we get older we drift from one subject to another (73-year-old woman, Spain).

Being unable to manage and control daily life could result in someone being 'reduced' as a person, as in one account where a woman described how her neighbour was made to be incontinent because of a lack of social service funding, and spoke of the impact of this on her self-respect and dignity. Similarly, having one's body exposed, or male nurses providing intimate care for older women, resulted in feelings of shame and humiliation which negatively affected the person's self-perception:

When I was in Hospital 2, I felt very embarrassed on the hoist and I used to say 'Can I cover myself up?' and they just pulled your nightie down over you, but the back view was wide open to anybody. … I was so embarrassed about that (68-year-old woman, UK).

Toileting practices often left older people feeling humiliated or embarrassed:

And you see again at night, they're short-staffed and she was told, 'Wet the bed, it's easier to change the bed than get the hoist' (65-year-old woman, UK).

This is where the pads come in, isn't it? It's easier to put pads and pants on people than to go and take them to the toilet. So people become incontinent when actually they needn't be (65-year-old woman, UK).

I've seen caregivers who didn't treat certain people in a dignified manner. Once one came in with a list to check who had to go to the toilet. People don't go to the toilet by list. They have to go when they need to. Someone asked the nurse to take them. She looked at the list and said, 'It's not your turn.' How do you like that? Does that person have dignity or not? That's not treating someone with dignity (78-year-old man, Spain).

Older participants cited numerous examples of how they or someone close to them had been the recipient of care that denied the dignity of identity. Often this resulted from insufficient staffing or resources so that old people ended up being 'warehoused', or as someone said, 'parked like cars', in overcrowded facilities where personalised care was impossible. Often, however, as in the examples cited above, staff attitudes were to blame, and most participants found it much easier to describe examples of care that detracted from their experience of dignity than to describe those which promoted it.

Dignified care
Care that enhanced the dignity of identity involved meaningful communication, kindness, politeness and a willingness to listen, together with the use of touch and human contact and a readiness to go the extra mile as this demonstrated the worth of the individual. When staff made special efforts to respond to the person as an individual, recognising their special needs, feelings of dignity were enhanced:

Well, if they wanted to talk to you about anything, or if you were upset, they talked to you privately and quietly and they would draw the curtains. The doctors always drew the curtains and if they wanted to look at your wound, they didn't just sort of throw the covers off you … they said 'Do you mind, can I have a look'? or if they brought someone different they would say, 'Do you think Dr whoever could have a look?' and they would introduce them. They didn't sort of barge in and take it for granted that you wouldn't mind what they were doing (70-year-old woman, UK).

Doctors and nurses were very kind to me in the C & M hospital and the head of department came too, even though it was at 11.p.m. I got injections and I sat in a chair all night (84-year-old woman, Slovakia).

[About a meeting with a nurse] *To allow a person plenty of time, to put things in order for us older people, with medicine and how we are feeling and everything. It was terrific. I can give this as an example of really dignified behaviour* (73-year-old male, Sweden).

And they touch them. Physical contact is very important. That person becomes closer through physical contact. A bond is established (73-year-old woman, Spain).

Thus the dignity of identity was crucially important to older people and was most likely to be at threat through contact with health and social care providers.

These three 'subjective' types of dignity are bound up with the everyday experiences of individuals and an absence of any of them may be felt as invisibility, shame, humiliation, degradation or embarrassment. The fourth type of dignity identified in the model is universal in nature.

6.2.4 Human dignity
This type of dignity was referred to by participants through reference to the inherent worth of human beings, or by appeals to human rights. For older participants, being

human represented an intrinsic dignity. Statements such as *treat me as a person, every human being has dignity,* and *everyone should be treated as an individual* were used by older people to describe human dignity:

Being recognised as a fellow human being (older person, Ireland).

These ideas were also commonly expressed by both young and middle-aged adults:

I've been trying to think of an all-embracing definition of dignity and it's very difficult. But the nearest I can think of is being treated with recognition of your rights as a human being (60-year-old man, UK).

Professional participants also acknowledged this type of dignity, and statements such as *we are dealing with human matters as well as human beings* indicated that health and social care workers recognised the universal nature of human dignity:

They are all important 'cos they are not a piece of meat that you can put from one place to another. They are humans – they have feelings (nursing home care assistant, UK).

As I see it, human dignity has a lot to do with the idea that the individual should be treated with dignity. And that rests upon our idea of human dignity: whether I am blind, deaf, suffer from dementia, am seriously ill or just old – I have human dignity (male physician, Sweden).

The right to freedom and autonomy was also a common theme in relation to this type of dignity. Despite their advancing years, older participants still wanted to retain control over their lives for as long as possible:

I know you are getting older and everybody lives a lot longer but you still want to be your own person, don't you? You don't want to be pushed around … (84-year-old woman, UK)

And then I also noticed, and this I hadn't noticed before, letters and decisions could arrive from authorities and they were not signed – nobody was responsible. Decisions had been taken, concerning me, without me taking part … who is representing me, acting in my place – who am I? (66-year-old woman, Sweden).

In particular, older people wanted to exercise choice about care alternatives. This was particularly so when a move into residential care was being considered and many participants found the thought of being forced into a care home particularly abhorrent.

One thing I have noticed here is that most people I know didn't come by their own decision. At one moment in their life, independent of their age and independent of being fit or not … it has been their family, their close relatives, their children who decided for them (83-year-old woman, France).

Those who have to go to one, to a nursing home, go to a barracks, eh? You have to be up at 8, breakfast at 10 … (90-year-old man, Spain).

Gaining patient consent, listening to their views, gaining their cooperation and allowing older people to experience some control and choice were all seen by professionals as ways of acknowledging the person's right to autonomy, which was seen as fundamental to maintaining their dignity.

To meet a person is to respect that she makes choices when she can make them. That she can ask and I respect her wishes. To respect her is also to give her a maximum of information so that she can make a choice and not to decide instead of her, because it is faster and it is easier for me to do so (female nursing assistant, France).

All her life, this person had been psychologically abused. Because this was a person who had never been good for anything and she was scorned in front of others. She was incapable of participating in a group. And then she was offered the opportunity and she managed to establish herself and began to communicate with the rest of the people. When it was over she came up to me and thanked me. Because it was the first time in her entire life that she had been treated with dignity, that she had been listened to, that she was able to explain her feelings and no one had expressed doubt about them … (female social work lecturer, Spain).

It is the simple things again that makes all the difference, like when you are getting a resident up in the morning, to give them the choice of what they would like to wear, what would you like to put on you today, as opposed to just pulling something over their head (female staff nurse, Ireland).

Young and middle-aged adults also believed that the rights to freedom, to choice, and to exercise control over one's life, were essential to maintaining human dignity. Even when concerns about the particular choices that older people may make were raised, many participants claimed that the 'right to choose' was more important to maintaining dignity than the appropriateness of the choice, and interesting debates about risk and older age often ensued.

Well, that's dignity isn't it, when you know your own mind and you want to choose things for yourself, and we don't want people to choose for us, do we? If you're dignified it's when you choose on your own, you have the freedom of choice to choose which direction your life takes. I don't see why that should change (52-year-old man, UK).

Even if the choice is inappropriate (50-year-old woman, UK).

It's your choice to make. It's still your choice to make. It's a free society. If you don't hurt anybody it's your choice to make. … That's where dignity comes in. Dignity is freedom of choice, do what you wish (52-year-old man, UK).

As well as autonomy and the right to exercise choice, equality was frequently mentioned as an important part of dignity. For older people, being treated as an equal, regardless of age, was important:

And there we are, everybody – we are all human beings (79-year-old man, Sweden).

Dignity exists when there are no differences, everyone is treated the same (82-year-old woman, Spain)

Dignity is not making any difference in the way you approach people because of their age. Treat them as an equal and as a person (81-year-old woman, UK).

Similarly, the notion of equality was frequently mentioned by professionals as a way to provide a dignified care.

An important attitude that there must be toward dignity is this one of 'between equals'. How do we position ourselves before the person? We position ourselves above them. And the key to respecting the person is to position yourself as an equal (female nurse, Spain).

I did indeed, yes, I guess what I mean is to meet them on equal terms or to meet people on equal terms and to talk about older people as a group feels a bit strange so it is just an equal meeting really and whatever you get you deal with it at the time, I mean you don't treat them in a certain way because they are older and equally you don't not treat them in a certain way because they are older, so I guess it is about an equality of meeting (female research nurse, UK).

6.3 Discussion

According to all participants, dignified care was empowering, courteous and capable of meeting individual needs, while undignified care was brutal, humiliating, narrow in focus, reliant on routine, made the person invisible and disempowered them. Participants also highlighted the barriers to dignified care which they believed exist in many European health and social care systems. These barriers included:

- Staff shortages and increased workloads.
- A lack of resources, together with impoverished environments, meant that even the most basic requirements were lacking.
- Managerialism and 'economic' approaches had shifted the focus on to getting the work done rather than providing personalised care.
- Emotional care was not high on institutional agendas and sometimes was even frowned upon.
- The emphasis on tasks that encouraged routine approaches to care could result in staff forgetting that they were dealing with people.
- Inappropriate attitudes on the part of some staff were also acknowledged.
- Lack of education, training and guidance on dignified care.

This study is the first attempt to explore comparative understandings, in terms both of participant groups and of nationalities, of the experiences of dignity in the lives of older people. Concerns on the part of researchers that participants would find it difficult to discuss dignity or that it would have little meaning to them were unfounded. None of the participants expressed any problems in speaking about dignity, and for older people in particular it was very relevant and salient to their lives. However, a number of methodological limitations are acknowledged. Despite efforts to include a broad spectrum of participants, there was a predominance of women in all of the focus groups, although this might reflect the demography both of the older populations and the health and social care occupations. The possible over-representation of women might also reflect either a specific interest in dignity or research in general, or it may be that women are more likely to take part in focus groups (Owen 2001). The study was based on participants' accounts and although it was not complemented by observational evidence (Mills et al. 1994) it confirms overall findings from research carried out in other contexts of care (Baldock & Haddow 2002). Holding focus groups at different sites and in different contexts increases the likelihood of identifying different and divergent discourses as well as enhancing reliability and validity (Kidd & Parshall 2000). However, despite this diversity there was a notable pattern of consistency within the findings. There was also considerable concurrence between the model of dignity and participants' accounts.

Rather than being a 'useless' concept which 'means no more than respect for persons or their autonomy' (Macklin 2003, p. 1419) dignity appeared to be a rich and salient concept for participants in this study. The participants believed that being treated with dignity was particularly important for older people and although the concept of dignity was sometimes difficult to capture, all participants could describe its various dimensions and were able to discuss at length the situations in which it might be threatened.

Participants' discourse suggested that the notion of dignity was of importance to ordinary people and that it allowed them to articulate their concerns about health and social care systems as well as with wider aspects of life. The theoretical model developed within the project should perhaps be refined to take account of the fact that most people appealed to dignity, not when they felt dignified, which to some extent is taken for granted, but rather when they felt that their dignity was being challenged or undermined. Older people in particular found it easier to recount situations or circumstances which threatened their dignity than those in which their dignity was enhanced.

The various types of dignity were relevant to most participants to a greater or lesser degree. For older adults the key element was the dignity of identity, although the dignity of merit and the dignity of moral stature were also discussed. Professionals also recognised the importance of the dignity of merit and the dignity of identity in relation to older people. Younger and middle-aged adults also discussed each type of dignity, displaying a considerable understanding of the needs and circumstances of many older people and the factors which impact most severely on their lives. All participants recognised the importance of human dignity (*Menschenwürde*) and that everyone, regardless of age, was equally deserving of this type of dignity. All participants recognised this as a basic human right.

To experience dignity of merit an individual has to be recognised by society as having dignity and a major claim of many older people was that they are not recognised or valued in modern society, making this type of dignity difficult to experience. The dignity of merit was also discussed by young and middle-aged adults in terms of its impact on the individual's self-esteem and in relation to the impact of inadequate finances on social inclusion. Frequent references were made to the special merit that the 'wisdom' of old age ought to bring.

The dignity of merit, as well as the dignity of moral stature, raised important issues for many professionals. These participants indicated that working with older people is not regarded as highly as working in other specialties. Again this is indicative of an underlying ageism. Professionals also reported their frustration at being unable to live up to the moral and professional requirements of their role, due to a lack of resources, under-staffing or inadequate care environments.

The dignity of moral stature was also of relevance to older adults, where it was frequently expressed in terms of appropriate behaviours, especially in difficult or offensive circumstances, such as being ridiculed or humiliated.

For older adults, it was, however, the dignity of identity which was most relevant. In the context of health and social care older people complained of being ignored, of being treated as objects, of having their need for privacy insufficiently recognised, of being humiliated and ridiculed and of inappropriate forms of address being used. The neglect of privacy impacted on the dignity of identity and centred on various situations involving toileting, intimate care being delivered by members of the opposite sex, especially in the case of older women, or being moved on a hoist with intimate body parts on display. In terms of dignity, what is at stake in such situations is the person's ability to control their relationships with others by maintaining the difference between public and private space and ensuring that necessary but embarrassing functions are carried out in private space. Although professionals frequently condemned such practices, they claimed that it was the context of care that sometimes made them unavoidable. For example, a male nurse may be the only person available to provide intimate care to an older woman. Clearly, issues related to dignity are not only about professional practice, but also reflect the resources and organisational structures within which these people work. Indignity may be as much a result of the institutional situation as of the callousness of an individual professional.

A similar point arises from the problem of how to address an older patient. Many older participants complained that they disliked the use of first names or pet names, like 'love' or 'dear', although some did recognise this as an attempt to be friendly. For many professionals, the use of a familiar name was part of a deliberate attempt to put the person at ease. Ironically, the indignity occurs not through an intentional act of humiliation or even thoughtlessness, but rather through a failure of communication (Woolhead et al. 2006). This may not be a matter of different generational cultures, but perhaps a reflection of the difference between the culture of the professional and that of the patient. This highlights the need for professional guidance and education as well as the resources to enable professionals to reflect on their practice and on the impact of their actions on those in their care.

Specifically, individuals felt undignified when their adult competence was compromised through illness and disability or by the actions of others. For many people the language of dignity appears to play an important role in protesting against feelings of humiliation, embarrassment and exclusion and the widespread stereotyping of older people which leads to institutional ageism (Ray et al. 2006).

Societal perceptions about the need for care, especially on an ongoing basis, appear to have acquired evaluative connotations so that requiring care appears to threaten the experience of dignity and not requiring care appears to have become a measure of individual dignity. Providing continuing care for older people is generally seen as routine and relatively undemanding, requiring only basic training, and Thompson (1995) argues that this is not simply a reflection of a lack of understanding, but instead suggests a more deeply ingrained negative and dismissive attitude towards older people, resulting in ageism, dehumanisation and a denial of dignity.

Population ageing and diminishing resources have resulted in many older people being required to pay for some or all of their care, being denied access to a number of treatments or experiencing cuts in services. For many, this subjection to unequal treatment is viewed as another way in which they are devalued, resulting in a loss of dignity as it prevents individuals from telling meaningful narratives about their lives or articulating their self-worth. This perceived lack of justice in health and social care thus amounts to indignity.

Rather than being seen as unproductive and a drain on resources, older people wanted to be appreciated for what they had achieved in their lives, and the contribution they had made to family and society. For professionals also, public recognition of their special skills was important.

Acknowledgement of individuality was an important part of the dignity of personal identity. Being recognised as someone with a history and relationships, someone who had once been where their carers were today, was important. Thus being treated in ways that were sympathetic to their personal history was essential to being treated with dignity. It was also necessary to take account of the vulnerabilities brought about by ageing and chronic illness and of the need for interdependence rather than focusing on dependence. Although the exercise of individual autonomy was an important element of experiencing dignity, an exclusive emphasis on individual autonomy, such as has been a tendency in health care ethics and has impacted on practice in health and social care services, could have negative consequences.

Pullman (1999) argues that to focus solely on considerations of autonomy assumes that the highest good is to maintain independence, and that dependence is a harm. He states that such a focus results in automatic failure for both the older person and those providing care when autonomy or independence cannot be restored. While for the majority of older people who are not frail the primacy of autonomy may be rightly placed, for many, the reality is that they will become more dependent and require increasingly extensive care.

We need therefore to consider the impact of such a focus, especially on the most severely dependent people. Too great an emphasis on autonomy can lead to such people being viewed as something less than human and therefore of less moral significance, as identified by both van Hooft et al. (1995) and Pullman (1999). Instead, we should acknowledge that even the most severely incapacitated person, such as someone in the final stages of dementia, still has moral worth despite being incapable of exercising any autonomy. Just existing as a human being confers a fundamental value (human dignity, *Menschenwürde*), and therefore demands our moral attention. It is also important to highlight that although it may not always be possible to promote autonomy, it is always possible to give care that enhances dignity. Indeed, we can violate a person's dignity if we set unrealistic goals in relation to autonomy.

When attention is refocused on the dignity of frail older people, all of their interests are protected even though their autonomy and the possibility of experiencing dignity may be lost. Such a shift of direction would also require that the dignity of the care provider is similarly considered and caring itself would acquire a greater moral value, as its intrinsic worth would be more readily apparent. As Pullman (1999) identifies, interdependence and the common dignity we all share as human beings should be what is emphasised, together with the humanity of both the cared-for and the caregiver.

It is a depressing indication that so many participants expressed the opinion that a life that was dependent must also lack dignity and therefore it is little wonder that care-giving for the frail and dependent is seen as inferior to more high-tech specialisms.

Ultimately, it is respect for human dignity or *Menschenwürde* which reflects our humanity and demonstrates our care and concern for frail older people such as those who are at the end of their life or those with severe dementia and it is our response to their inherent moral worth that enhances and expresses our own dignity. The words of one older participant echo this sentiment perfectly:

> *It is in care that human dignity is consolidated. You feel more valued, when someone takes care of you. It is a demonstration of love and that gives dignity.*

6.4   Conclusion

This study has provided evidence that the language of dignity plays an important role in the lives of older people and the recent emphasis on dignity in current health and social policy may be timely, although it might be undermined by policies that promote performance targets which encourage throughput and access but reduce the time available for care. This may serve to maintain rather than combat institutional ageism. Meanwhile professionals can do much to safeguard the dignity of service-users by addressing aspects of their practice that threaten the dignity of identity of older people and also by taking appropriate opportunities to use their professional status to secure the resources necessary to provide dignified care.

Acknowledgements

The Dignity and Older Europeans project was funded by the European Commission, DG Research, Directorate E: Biotechnology, Agriculture and Food, under FP5, Quality of Life Programme (Contract QLG6-CT-2001-00888). We thank all the study participants for giving their time and information.

References

Arino-Blasco, S., Tadd, W. & Boix-Ferrer, J.A. (2005) Dignity and older Europeans: the voice of professionals. *Quality in Ageing: Policy, Practice and Research*, **6**, 30–36.
Baggott, R., Allsop, J. & Jones, K. (2005) *Speaking for Patients and Carers: Health Consumer Groups and the Policy Process*. Palgrave, Basingstoke.
Baldock, J. & Haddow, J. (2002) Self-talk versus needs-talk. *Quality in Ageing: Policy, Practice and Research*, **3**, 42–48.

Bayer, T., Tadd, W. & Krajcik, S. (2005) Dignity and older Europeans: voices of older people. *Quality in Ageing: Policy, Practice and Research*, **6**, 22–29.

Beach, M.C., Sugarman, J., Johnson, R.L., Arbelaez, J.J., Duggan, P.S. & Cooper, L.A. (2005) Do patients treated with dignity report higher satisfaction, adherence and receipt of preventive care? *Annals of Family Medicine*, **3**, 331–338.

Bensink, G.W., Godbey, K.L., Marshall, M.J. & Yarandi, H.N. (1992) Institutionalized elderly: relaxation, locus of control, self-esteem. *Journal of Gerontological Nursing*, **18**, 30–38.

Bloor, M., Frankland, J., Thomas, M. & Robson, K. (2000) *Focus Groups in Social Research*. Sage, London.

Brazinová, A., Janská, E. & Jurkovi, R. (2004) Implementation of patients' rights in the Slovak Republic. *Eubios Journal of Asian and International Bioethics*, **14**, 90–91.

Brillhart, B. & Johnson, K. (1997) Motivation and the coping process of adults with disabilities: a qualitative study. *Rehabilitation Nursing*, **22**, 249–252; 255–256.

Calnan, M. & Tadd, W. (2005) Dignity and older Europeans: methodology. *Quality in Ageing: Policy, Practice and Research*, **6**, 10–16.

Calnan, M., Almond, S. & Smith, N. (2003) Ageing and public satisfaction with the health service: an analysis of recent trends. *Social Science and Medicine*, **57**, 757–762.

CHI (2003) *Investigation into Matters Arising from Care on Rowan Ward, Manchester Mental Health and Social Care Trust*. Commission for Health Improvement. HMSO, London.

Council of Europe (1997) *Convention for the Protection of Human Rights and Dignity of the Human Being With Regard to the Application of Biology and Medicine*. Convention on Human Rights and Medicine. European Treaty Series **164**, Council of Europe, Strasbourg.

DH (2000) *The NHS Plan*. Department of Health HMSO, London.

DH (2001a) *National Service Framework for Older People*. Department of Health. HMSO, London.

DH (2001b) *Caring for Older People: A Nursing Priority*. Department of Health. HMSO, London.

DH (2006a) *A New Ambition for Old Age*. Department of Health. HMSO, London.

DH (2006b) *Dignity in Care Initiative*. Department of Health, London. Available online at http://www.dh.gov.uk/en/SocialCare/Socialcarereform/Dignityincare/index.htm [Accessed 3 August 2006].

Edgar, A. (2004) A response to Nordenfelt's 'The varieties of dignity'. *Health Care Analysis*, **12**, 83–89.

Gallagher, A. & Seedhouse, D. (2002) Dignity in care: the views of patients and relatives. *Nursing Times*, **98**, 38–40.

Gilleard, C. & Higgs, P. (2000) *Culture and Ageing: Self, Citizen and the Body*. Prentice Hall, Harlow.

Glendinning, C., Clarke, S., Hare, P., Kotchetkova, I., Maddison, J. & Newbronner, L. (2006) *Outcomes-Focused Services for Older People*. Social Care Institute for Excellence, London.

Haddock, J. (1996) Toward a further clarification of the concept 'dignity'. *Journal of Advanced Nursing*, **29**, 924–931.

HAS 2000 (1998) *Not Because They Are Old. Health*. Health Advisory Service, London.

ICN (2000) *Code of Ethics for Nurses*. International Council of Nurses, Geneva.

Jacelon, C. (2004) A concept analysis of dignity for older adults. *Journal of Advanced Nursing*, **48**, 76–83.

Keith, J., Fry, C.L. & Ikels, C. (1990) Community as context for successful aging. In: *The Cultural Context of Aging: Worldwide Perspectives*, (ed J. Sokolovsky), pp. 245–261. Bergin & Garvey, New York.

Kenny, T. (1990) Erosion of individuality in care of elderly people in hospital: an alternative approach. *Journal of Advanced Nursing*, **15**, 571–576.

Kidd, P.S. & Parshall, M. (2000) Getting the focus and the group: enhancing analytical rigor in focus group research. *Qualitative Health Research*, **10**, 293–308.

Kitzinger, J. (1995) Introducing focus groups. *British Medical Journal*, **311**, 299–302.

Kitzinger, J. (2000) Introducing focus groups. In: *Qualitative Research in Health Care* (ed. C. Pope & N. Maysm), pp. 20–29. BMJ Books, London.

Kitzinger, J. & Barbour, R. (1999). Introduction: the challenge and promise of focus groups. In: *Developing Focus Group Research* (ed R. Barbour & J. Kitzinger), pp. 1–20. Sage, London.

Levenson, R. (2002) *Auditing Age Discrimination*. King's Fund, London.

Macklin, R. (2003) Dignity is a useless concept. *BMJ*, **327**, 1419–20.

Mills, M., Davies, H. & Macrae, W. (1994) Care of dying patients in hospital. *BMJ*, **309**, 583–586.

MHSA (1997). *Health and Medical Services Act*. Law decided by the Riksdag 1996:786, Ministry of Health and Social Affairs, Stockholm.

NMC (2004) *Code of Professional Conduct*. Nursing and Midwifery Council, London.

Nordenfelt, L. (2003) Dignity and the care of the elderly. *Medicine, Health Care and Philosophy*, **6**, 103–110.

Nordenfelt, L. (2004) The varieties of dignity. *Health Care Analysis*, **12**, 69–81.

Nordenfelt, L. & Edgar, A. (2005) The four notions of dignity. *Quality in Ageing: Policy, Practice and Research*, **6**, 17–21.

Owen, S. (2001) The practical methodological and ethical dilemmas of conducting focus groups with vulnerable clients. *Journal of Advanced Nursing*, **26**, 652–658.

Pokorny, M.E. (1989) The Effects of Nursing Care on Human Dignity in the Critically Ill Adult. PhD thesis, University of Virginia, Maryland.

Pullman, D. (1999) The ethics of autonomy and dignity in long-term care. *Canadian Journal on Aging*, **18**, pp. 26–49.

Ranzijn, R., Keeves, J., Luszcz, M. & Feather, N.T. (1998) The role of self-perceived usefulness and competence in the self-esteem of elderly adults: confirmatory factor analysis of the Bachman Revision of Rosenberg's self-esteem scale. *Journal of Gerontology*, **53**, 96–104.

Ray, S., Sharp, E. & Abrams, D. (2006) *How Ageist is Britain? A Benchmark of Public Attitudes in Britain*. Age Concern, London.

Seedhouse, D. & Gallagher, A. (2002) Undignifying institutions. *Journal of Medical Ethics*, **28**, 368–372.

Shotton, L. & Seedhouse, D. (1998). Practical dignity in caring. *Nursing Ethics*, **5**, 246–255.

Söderberg, A., Gilje, F., & Norberg, A. (1997) Dignity in situations of ethical difficulty intensive care. *Intensive Critical Care Nursing*, **13**, 135–144.

Spiegelberg, H. (1970) Human dignity: a challenge to contemporary philosophy. In: *Human Dignity: This Century and the Next* (eds R. Gotesky and E. Laszlo), pp. 39–64. Gordon & Breach Science, New York.

Stratton, D. & Tadd, W. (2005) Dignity and older people: the voice of society. *Quality in Ageing – Policy, Practice and Research*, **6**, 37–45.

Strauss, A. & Corbin, J. (1998) *Basics of Qualitative Research*. Sage, Thousand Oaks, CA.

Tadd, W. & Bayer, A. (2001) Dignity as a feature of complaints by elderly people. *Age and Ageing*, **30**, 40.

Tadd, W., Dieppe, P. & Bayer, T. (2002) Dignity in health care: reality or rhetoric. *Reviews in Clinical Gerontology*, **12**, 1–4.

Thompson, N. (1995) *Age and Dignity: Working with Older People*. Arena, Aldershot.

UNO (1948) *The Universal Declaration of Human Rights.* General Assembly resolution 217 A (111), 10 December, Office of the High Commissioner for Human Rights, United Nations Organization, Geneva.

van Hooft, S., Gillam, L. & Byrnes, M. (1995) *Facts and Values: An Introduction to Critical Thinking for Nurses.* Maclennan & Petty, Sydney.

WAG (2007) *Action Taken to Improve Respect and Dignity of Older People.* Welsh Assembly Government. Available online at http://new.wales.gov.uk/topics/health/news/respect/?lang=en [accessed 23 January 2008]

Walker, A. (1999) Older people and health services: the challenge of empowerment. In: *Health and Exclusion: Policy and Practice in Health Provision* (eds M. Purdy and D. Banks), pp. 158–178, Routledge, London.

Walsh, K. & Kowanko, I. (2002) Nurses' and patients' perceptions of dignity. *International Journal of Nursing Practice*, **8**, 143–151.

Webb, C. Kevern, J. (2001) Focus groups as a research method: a critique of some aspects of their use in nursing research. *Journal of Advanced Nursing*, **33**, 798–805.

Woolhead, G., Calnan, M., Dieppe, P. & Tadd, W. (2003) Dignity in older age: what do older people in the United Kingdom think? *Age and Ageing*, **33**, 165–170.

Woolhead, G., Tadd, W., Boix-Ferrer, A.J. et al. (2006) 'Tu' or 'vous'? A European qualitative study of dignity and communication with older people in health and social care settings. *Patient Education and Counseling*, **61**, 363–71.

7. A Dignified Death and Identity-Promoting Care

Britt-Marie Ternestedt

Introduction

Approximately 92 000 people die in Sweden every year, most of whom are aged 75 or over. The trend is to transfer the care of dying patients from the hospital to the home. An underlying assumption is that care in one's own home usually improves the chances of a dignified or good death. Those who live and die in sheltered accommodation are included in the term 'home'. For many people, a dignified or good death has been described as one that involves dying quickly, preferably in one's everyday environment and when asleep in one's own bed, as well as being mentally alert and maintaining control until the end. A dignified death has also been described as being associated with death from certain diseases and without unnecessary use of resources or extraordinary interventions (Rinell Hermansson 1990). However, most people will not die such a death. On the contrary, approximately 80% will die slowly, which means gradual deterioration and increasing dependence on others. The terms 'dignified death' and 'good death' can be considered limiting in that they tend to make one think about the actual moment of death. The most common meaning is, however, far wider and includes both the preceding period of dying and the hours immediately following the death when the body is taken care of.

This chapter will illuminate what dying people describe as a meaningful life and a dignified death, and what they regard as threats to these ideals. The chapter is based on results from studies carried out by two different research groups. One of these groups was formed in the early 1990s in connection with the planning and establishment of a hospice unit and has to date focused mainly on the situation of cancer patients, their next of kin and staff. The second research group, known as the Home project, came into being in early 2000 and includes researchers from different disciplines. Empirical findings about how older people experience the final phase of life have been constantly reflected upon in relation to theoretical and philosophical terms. Conversely, the meanings of such terms have been analysed and compared with the empirical data. This book is to a great extent a result of this project. What the two groups have in common is that they focus on the meanings of dignity and a good death. This indicates that many of the sub-projects in both groups involved concepts such as dignity, auton-omy and quality of life. This chapter will focus particularly on the concept of dignity of identity.

In Chapter 2, Lennart Nordenfelt describes the concept of dignity of identity as 'the dignity we attach to ourselves as integrated and autonomous persons, persons with a history and persons with a future with all our relationships to other human beings'. In Chapter 4, Magnus Öhlander outlines the work involved in the care given to people with dementia to ensure that they retain as much of their identity as possible. The present chapter describes the continuous work that seriously ill and elderly people do, mainly by themselves, to maintain as much of their identity or self as possible until death. However, nurses and other carers have a major responsibility for promoting a dying person's possibilities of retaining as much of their identity or self as possible until the moment of death. In the literature, identity and self are often used as synonyms. However, one distinction is that identity involves a sociological view of human beings and self reflects a more psychological perspective – how the person experiences them-self (see Chapter 5). In this chapter I have chosen to talk about identity in a way close to what Nordenfelt has called *dignity of identity* and my co-workers and I have named *maintained self-image*.

One point of departure in this chapter is a nursing perspective. A number of concepts are considered fundamental for both the practical performance of nursing care and nursing science, such as person, health and environment. The theoretical loading of these concepts depends on the perspective on the individual, including the view of human development and how knowledge is created. My view is that nursing science is at the point of intersection between the individual and society. In the practice of nursing, this means that the encounter between patient and nurse on an individual level reflects organisational and societal levels. Consequently, palliative care nursing does not take place in a vacuum but is shaped in a certain society at a particular point in time. This raises the question of whether societal-level values expressed in policy docu-ments on health and medical care are in agreement with the way in which care is organised and carried out. For example, is palliative care available to everyone irrespec-tive of place of residence, age and diagnosis? Or is there a gap between the expressed ideals and the opportunities for carers to provide such care? Several studies indicate the latter (Whitaker 2004; Goodridge et al. 2005; Seymour et al. 2005; Jakobsson et al. 2006; Connor 2007/2008; Dwyer 2008; Tadd & Calnan, this volume, Chapter 6). Western society applauds values such as youth, health, strength and autonomy, but disease, dying, death and dependence threaten these values and for this reason easily become invisible. Despite the totality of individual death, it is often swept under the carpet. During their final year of life, people have a very great need of assistance irrespective of age. There are some indications that older people and those with diseases other than cancer are often discriminated against in terms of access to palliative care (WHO 2004a; Dwyer 2008). The document *Better Palliative Care for Older People* (WHO 2004a) considers this injustice as an expression of ageism and states that the deficiency should be rem-edied by the implementation of palliative care in all areas of care, not least in nursing homes, where many people spend their last days. It is reasonable to assume that this would have a positive impact on many people's everyday life and experience of dignity.

7.1 A dignified or good death

The concept of dignity is employed in many health-care policy documents, but its meaning is rarely clarified. Dignity can, among other things, reflect both an attitude towards other people and towards oneself (self-respect). There are different views and descriptions of what is appropriate or inappropriate in order for the final phase of life to be described as dignified. In research, there are a number of concepts that are often used synonymously with a dignified death, for example an 'appropriate death' (Weisman & Kastenbaum 1968; Weisman 1974), a 'good death' (McNamara et al. 1995; Payne et al. 1996; Lloyd 2004), a 'peaceful death' (Callahan 1993; Snyder 1994; Meier et al. 1997) and a 'healthy death' (Russel & Sander 1998; cf. Fryback 1993). Common to all these concepts is the fact that they indicate values that should be promoted at the end of life, such as retaining one's self-image and integrity, self-respect, self-determination and preserving social relationships, the meanings of which can be summarised as preserving identity. Relieving the patient's suffering and symptoms is always a central concern. To a certain extent, the descriptions of a dignified death and its synonyms reveal the need of the dying person to speak about and summarise his or her life. Narratives based on the individual's biography are often characterised as bolstering the sense of identity and the ability to become reconciled both with one's past life and with the fact that life will soon come to a close (see Chapter 8). Accordingly, it is important that the dying person is seen as someone with a specific life history and as more than an objective body. The subjective and lived body also needs to be held in respect (see Chapter 3). Our own research, based on dying people's narratives, has shown that a dignified death means being allowed to be the person one is until the end. Many people also find it essential to feel that they belong to a group, which can consist of their family as well as other nursing home residents and/or staff. Being someone in relation to others is central. Dying people have also mentioned they have a need to provide care, not only to receive care from others. Being able to both provide and receive care, as well as sharing the joys and concerns of everyday life, creates meaning. However, very old or dying people are sometimes, out of misdirected concern, deprived of tasks that provide meaning. Being seen as a person with experiences and being remembered as someone is of central importance even at the very end of life, and perhaps particularly then. This will be apparent from examples provided later in the chapter.

The modern hospice movement founded by Dame Cicely Saunders has had a major impact on care in the final phase of life. The care philosophy on which St Christopher's Hospice was built has spread all over the world and has come to mean a great deal to dying people, their families and also to staff who care for seriously ill and dying patients. Saunders stressed at an early stage that care, education and research were the main components that made it possible to reach the goal of hospice philosophy. Today, about 40 years later, this goal remains highly relevant. Although much has been achieved, much remains to be done worldwide (Clark 2007/2008; Twycross 2007/2008).

All in all, modern hospice philosophy can be described as a paradigm shift from a paternalistic to a holistic perspective, where every patient is considered a unique person with the right of self-determination, even when they are dying. Hospice philosophy emphasises the importance of providing the family with support during a difficult time, with the aim of promoting the quality of life of all family members.

The growth of hospice care can be seen as an expression of societal change in line with postmodern trends that, for example, highlight autonomy, individualism and pluralism. The United Kingdom and the United States have a tradition of different forms of hospice care. This tradition does not exist in Sweden, where for many years there was opposition to the development of such care. Instead, in the late 1970s the goal was that the pervading ideal of all care of the dying, irrespective of where it was provided, should be close to that of hospice philosophy, a goal that was not achieved. Hospice care is thus a relatively recent phenomenon in Sweden. The first hospices were established in the early 1980s and almost invariably provide home and in-patient care, the latter often in a small unit. Day care is extremely rare.

In recent years the concept of palliative care has gradually replaced that of hospice care. The most common definition of palliative care is that of the World Health Organization (WHO). Palliative care has been defined as an approach that improves the quality of life of patients and their families facing the problem associated with life-threatening illness, through the prevention and relief of suffering by means of early identification, an impeccable assessment and treatment of pain and other problems, physical, psychosocial and spiritual (WHO 2004b). The WHO document also states that

> Palliative care provides relief from pain and other distressing symptoms, affirms life and regards dying as a normal process, and intends neither to hasten nor to prolong death. Palliative care integrates the psychological and spiritual aspects of patient care and offers a support system to help patients live as actively as possible until death. It also offers a support system to help the family cope during the patient's illness and in their own bereavement. Using a team approach, palliative care addresses the needs of patients and their families, including bereavement counselling if necessary. It enhances quality of life and may positively influence the course of the illness (WHO 2004b, p. 14).

As mentioned earlier, it is acknowledged that not everyone has the same access to good palliative care, in particular old people and those with illnesses other than cancer. In recent years several conventional care units have changed their designation to palliative care units. Whether they adhere to palliative care philosophy has not been investigated to any great extent, and research is needed in this area.

7.2 Being allowed to be the person one is and to decide for oneself

In Chapter 4 of this volume, Öhlander focuses on the work of promoting dignity of identity in the everyday life of people with dementia. The following is a description of how one person with advanced cancer fought to maintain his self-determination for as long as possible. He wanted to live his own life in accordance with his values. The brief summary will make it clear that this man, David, had to stand up for himself in various ways. His efforts can be said to constitute a continuous attempt to maintain as much of his identity and self as possible, as illustrated by, for example, the form of care he chose for the final phase of life.

David was 75 years old and had a long working life behind him. He started work on a farm at the age of 14. By the time he retired he was a well-respected foreman of an industrial company. An important part of David's identity was his involvement with the Church of Sweden. He had been a widower for five years. He had two adult children and six grandchildren. He was convalescing after an operation during which it was established that he had inoperable stomach cancer. The events described below took place at the time when David was to be discharged from a short-term facility. Up to that point he had been cared for there for about a month, and he had felt safe and happy.

The setting for the meeting is David's private room and David is in bed. He looks remarkably well, despite his serious illness. The white hospital gown with a purple scarf tied around his thin neck suits him. A couple of weeks ago he was informed that he has a form of cancer that can be neither operated on nor treated. The cancer has spread to the peritoneum. Just a few months ago he had felt well and fairly fit. He had gone for long walks almost every day, often with a female friend. He had enjoyed life. Then everything changed, food no longer tasted good, he found it difficult to eat, developed stomach pain and lost a huge amount of weight. His clothes became too loose and one day he plucked up courage and went to see the doctor. He was immediately referred to an emergency hospital for an operation, but it was too late. David was to be discharged a few days after the operation, but he refused to go. He was not ready! His obstinacy, combined with charm, was successful and he was given a bed in a short-term care facility. Persistent asking pays off in the end, as he said himself. He did not want to give up something that was beneficial for him. But the respite period was now over, and he was to be discharged in order to make room for another patient. He reluctantly accepted that there was no other alternative. He now lay in bed and awaited the arrival of the 'planners', as he called the nurse and the care manager (a social worker) who were to carry out the discharge planning. His two middle-aged children sat on chairs in a corner of the room. They had chosen this position in order to allow the planners to sit beside their Dad's bed. They waited with a certain amount of tension. What would happen? How much responsibility would they have to assume for looking after their father? And how were they to manage to care for him in the midst of all their other responsibilities? Many questions were going around in their heads. At the same time as they worried about practical matters, they experienced grief, as they understood that David was close to death. Against this background, their thoughts about practical matters were felt to be inappropriate.

With a light tap on the door, the care manager carrying a file and the nurse with medical responsibility, notepad in hand, enter the room. They greet his children with a brief nod and go up to David and one of them says: 'Now we shall deal with the care planning'. David smiles warmly and starts to raise himself up to a sitting position in order to talk and, when upright, says slowly in his weak voice but in a self-assured manner: 'Yes, and I shall be the chairman!' There is silence, nobody says anything. David carefully reaches for the notepad and pen that lie on the bedside table. Then he says: 'What is it about? Let me know, tell me!' 'Yes', says the nurse, 'we think that you should receive assistance from HHC when you get home. Everything will be fine.' 'H H C', David repeats slowly, and he writes the letters in the note pad. He pronounces them again: 'H H C, what sort of an organisation is that?' The nurse explains that the letters stand for Hospital-linked Home Care and goes on to describe how good the home care is in general and how appropriate it would be for David. David listens politely. The nurse continues (with the best of intentions): 'I'll phone you tomorrow and we can arrange a time when someone will visit you at home and register you for the home care service.' David answers in a pleasant but firm manner: 'I don't think so, it needs some thought. This is all new to me and I have to consider it, it's happening too quickly.' There is a long silence and after a while David adds: 'Let's say that I'll phone you if I want home care. I need to think about it.' After a further attempt to convince him, the care manager and the nurse leave the room without having achieved anything.

The silence is heavy in the room for a while, until David breaks it and says to his children: 'I want my freedom, I don't want to be registered in my own home, I want to try to manage myself or come up with another solution' (Ternestedt 2007).

David was discharged and thanks to his friends and his children he was able to feel free in his own home for a few months. He lived as independently as he could within the boundaries imposed by his condition. He then took the initiative and obtained hospice care for the final weeks of his life, where he continued to set the pace. He enjoyed himself there and he almost felt that his life was luxurious. As long as he was physically able to do so, he passed the time playing the keyed fiddle in his room. He sometimes brought the instrument into the day room, where he played for guests and relatives. He also played with the other musicians at the hospice ward's midsummer celebration. What surprised the people around him, not least his children, was the fact that, despite a relatively short period of illness, he was reconciled to the fact that he would soon die.

One can question whether David's story romanticises dying and the encounter with death. I would say that David's death represents one of death's many faces. To a great extent it mirrors David as a person, and one could say that he had the 'good fortune' to be afflicted by a form of cancer of which the symptoms can more or less be relieved (he expressed this himself, as his wife had experienced a very difficult death). This improved his chances of being independent in the highly dependent situation in which he found himself. In spite of all the limitations, he felt free. David could be said to have maintained his identity and thus also his dignity right up to his death.

The account of David will now be related to three perspectives on death which are usually described as the traditional, modern and late modern, also known as postmodern, death. These three perspectives can all be found in David's narrative, both implicitly and explicitly.

7.3 Death as a religious, medical and private event

Several social scientists, such as Tony Walter (1994) and Zygmunt Bauman (1992), have given interesting accounts of how our perspective on death can be understood in relation to contemporary societal values. Both describe how the view of death has changed over time in line with other changes in society, generally associated with different periods of societal development. Traditional death is often related to the values embraced by an agricultural society, modern death is mirrored by the values of an industrial society and postmodern death by the values that characterise present-day society. By analogy with such a time-related definition, death can also be described as a religious, medical or private family event, or as a combination of all three.

Tony Walter's descriptions of different perspectives on death and dying are characterised by how the view of death and its associated rituals change in line with societal changes. The three above-mentioned perspectives on death should be seen as typologies and simplifications of complex relationships in the Western world (Walter 1994; Ternestedt 2007). However, they clearly illustrate how values at the macro level are reflected at the meso and micro levels. A concrete example of this is the attitude towards the authorities and the context in which the dying and death take place. The three perspectives can be integrated in the identity of a single individual, and at the same time as one of them can be more dominant, which can be said to have been the case with David.

7.3.1 Traditional death

Looking back over the past hundred years provides a clear picture of how quickly society has changed and how differently people in the Western world lived a hundred years ago in comparison with today. In Sweden the average life expectancy was low, child mortality was high and few people survived to become what we call today 'the oldest old'. The disease panorama was different. Knowledge of medications and medical treatment was limited. Epidemics were frequent and the lack of, for example, antibiotics meant that the time between the onset of illness and death was short. Traditional death is usually described as a natural part of a person's life in an agricultural society. Compared to today, death was very much a part of everyday life and thereby a social event. Both birth and death took place in the home (Walter 1994). During this period, the role of the church was much more important in everyday life in Sweden than it is today. Many people had religious faith and believed in a life after death. When someone fell ill, their soul had to have peace and quiet and thus the priest was often the first to be summoned. Clergymen and the church, as opposed to doctors and natural science, were the authorities on which people pinned their expectations. Against this background, traditional death was seen as a religious event. One of the characteristics of traditional death was the associated rituals that dictated the way in which mourning should take place. Death and mourning were visible and not swept under the carpet. The mourners often wore black clothing or armbands for a certain period of time, which gave them a measure of identity. Furthermore, death and mourning involved neighbours and others and were thus a social events.

The perspective that corresponds to traditional death, albeit in a slightly modified form, is still valid today. Although secularised, like many other Western countries, Sweden is a multicultural and pluralistic society and thus even today death remains very much a religious event. If we return to David, we find that he had a deep-rooted religious faith. He had a kind of inner peace and did not talk very much about his spiritual or existential needs. He lived his life, carried out everyday chores and passed away, feeling secure because of trust in God, himself and his surroundings. Reliance and trust were strongly integrated in David's identity.

7.3.2 Death as a medical event: modern death

Social scientists have described how agricultural society was gradually replaced by what we usually call modern society. Industrialisation and the growth of modern society changed the perspective on death. The standard of living became higher, child mortality decreased and the average life expectancy gradually increased. Medical and scientific advances contributed to curing illnesses that had previously been fatal. Death moved from everyday life into the hospital, where it became the concern of the medical profession. Concurrently with medical and scientific advances, death was more and more regarded as a failure. In other words, religion, the church and the clergy lost authority and were mainly replaced by medical science and the doctor. In literature, hospitals were described as the temples of the new era. This change in perspective and the possibilities of receiving care can be regarded as a paradigm shift. The focus of care changed from peace for the soul to treatment for the body. For the individual hospital patient, this sometimes meant that, when nothing more could be done in terms of treatment, the professionals lost interest. There is much anecdotal evidence of the rounds passing by the dying patient's bed. As a result, many dying patients received care that was far too passive and surrounded by silence. The dying patient came to personify death, and death was something to be avoided rather than addressed. A short time before death, the dying person was often moved to a private room. The main reason was not that they should be undisturbed and able to be with their family, but to avoid frightening or upsetting others. Other patients and visitors should be protected from having to confront death. Death became a medical event. The authority of the clergy and the church was replaced by that of doctors and medical science. As a result, dying, death and the associated rituals became professionalised. The family members perceived themselves as being of minor importance, as they were only allowed to visit the patient at fixed times. The rituals and routines were designed to suit the needs of the health-care system rather than those of the patient and family. A funeral industry that managed all practical funeral arrangements accordingly developed, which meant that 'ordinary' people became less and less involved in shaping the rituals associated with death. All in all, this has probably contributed to our reluctance to think about death and made us afraid of it.

In the late 1960s, the medical perspective was challenged by the modern hospice movement. The focus shifted from a medical to a holistic perspective on the human being. In my opinion, this development can be understood as an early postmodern current, which in Sweden is supported by the new Health and Medical Services Act emphasising patient autonomy.

Death as a medical event is still very much in evidence, something which many of us have experienced, whether as carers, patients or family members. The silence surrounding death has perhaps been somewhat reduced, although this is open to discussion. The literature reveals that the results of studies focused on openness to death are far from unambiguous. Several studies indicate, however, that many people want to be participants in their own care and informed about the prognosis of their disease, for example.

When this discussion was ongoing in the 1970s, the concept of truthfulness was often mentioned, as well as the fact that patients and their family members should be allowed to share the knowledge of health professionals. However, the discussion concerned being as truthful as possible and not the truth as such (as no one knows the definitive truth when it comes to a prognosis, for example). If we return to David, we can say that he had great confidence in medical science, but not blind faith. It is possible that David's trust in medical science prompted him to choose a hospice for the final days of his life, as he felt safe there and for this reason did not want home care or to die at home. He was surrounded by a social network that would probably have supported him to the very last minute, had he chosen to be cared for in his own home. What is interesting is that he was aware that this form of care existed, and knew what it meant. When informed that his cancer was incurable, he understood the implication and continued his life, perhaps more intensely than before. Information and participation were important to him and constituted the prerequisite for being able to prepare for the final phase of his life. Of course, for other individuals the scenario may be different. In the transition between modern and postmodern society, mainly psychiatrists, psychologists and a few nurses started to carry out scientific studies focusing on death. Nurses' studies included the patient's perspective on dying (Qvarnström 1978) as well as their own perspective on caring for seriously ill and dying patients for a relatively long period (Vachon 2001). It is important to remember that the duration of nursing care was much longer than it is today; for example, several months in a hospice ward was not unusual. The postmodern ideal is that all human beings should be allowed to approach death in their own fashion, irrespective of what that may imply.

7.3.3   Postmodern death: a private event

The concepts of late modern and postmodern are complex and the subject of ongoing discussion. Many social scientists have discussed the dialectics between postmodern and modern. The concepts are used to describe two historical eras. The term postmodernism has been employed to denote a radical shift between epochs, where the modern is left behind and the emergence of a qualitatively new societal system can be discerned. The term postmodern is sometimes used as a label for ambivalence, reflexivity and pluralism.

Ambivalence can be related to all options that a person faces in a society where traditions have weakened or become less important. Control and order are difficult to attain and, as Bauman (1992) states, human beings try to cope with this ambivalence in different ways. One way of avoiding ambivalence is to adopt the approach that it is possible to attain control and order despite the lack of a comprehensive perspective and clear-cut solutions. Another way is to recognise ambivalence at the cost of a stable identity. Bauman (1992) states that many people try to create balance in their daily life by shifting between these two approaches. Reflexivity influences the individual's life world and identity and means that even everyday life becomes the subject of analysis. Identity is not seen as natural and static but something that human beings themselves are to a great extent responsible for creating. It is not a question of creating a given identity, as postmodern human beings move in different situations and contexts, where they choose how to present themselves. Therefore, identity in postmodern society is usually described as fluid, and increased individualisation is noticeable. In that sense individuals are their own authority. To put it simply, human beings are free to choose their own lifestyle even when close to death. Death and dying are usually described as a project that each person is expected to stage him or herself, i.e. they construct their own death. In a sense, this is what David did. He exercised his self-determination to the very last moment within the framework of the dependence caused by the disease and the overall situation. He rejected expert advice that was incompatible with the way in which he wanted to live his final days.

Simply put, industrial society can be said to have been replaced by the information and consumer society, where the human being is more or less regarded as an independent actor. If the priest and doctor were previously regarded as authorities, a shift can now be seen towards the individual. This freedom constitutes a paradox, as it creates a demand for new experts and authorities: some examples are the media and different kinds of therapists. In a secularised society characterised by a lack of tradition, the absence of rituals and somebody whom one can trust may give rise to feelings of existential loneliness and emptiness at the individual level. This is especially true of death. A good or dignified death means one that is consistent with the dying person's values. This implies that the dying person is to be regarded as an authority in the sense that he is both capable of influencing and should be allowed to influence his own death. Today, many patients obtain information from the Internet in addition to that provided by doctors and health-care staff. A parallel can be drawn with giving birth, which in hospitals today has become more adapted to the needs of the woman and the family and has thus become a family event. Death is also gradually becoming a family event. Today, the patient and the family carers increasingly wish to participate in the planning of rituals surrounding death and dying, or to create their own rituals. It should be a matter of course to include patients and next of kin in the palliative team.

Various health-care policy documents give expression to the ideal of autonomy and freedom of choice at the societal level. As mentioned above, the home is considered to represent this ideal. The number of in-patient care beds has been reduced and the home care service expanded. An increasing number of people are now dying in their own home (although not always by their own choice). Thus death has more and more become a private event that takes place within the family sphere. This means a new and important role for family carers who want to influence and be involved in the care of the sick and dying person. The death of a family member may be their first encounter with death, which can make it difficult to know both one's own wishes and what it is possible to do. When it comes to promoting a dignified or good death, the dying person and the family are dependent upon the health professionals, sharing knowledge and informing them about what they think will happen. The family of today often differs from that of previous generations, as family members are more likely to live far away and family patterns are more complex. This requires new types of solutions to the problems that can arise when a family member is about to die. Postmodern death is characterised by pluralism and the absence of a ready template for a good or dignified death. The guiding principles are diversity and individualisation. A dignified or good death must always be seen in relation to the individual's lifestyle and outlook on life. It does not preclude the existence of common traits, although these can be laden with completely different values depending on the individual in question.

7.4 Extended identity close to death

According to the theory of human psychosocial development put forward by Erik Homburger Erikson and his wife Joan Erikson, the human being undergoes a life-long struggle to try to attain and maintain a stable self. The self is not something we casually adopt; on the contrary, it is deeply rooted in the person and must be constantly re-examined. It is developed in the interaction between biological, psychological, social and cultural processes, even at the end of life. In the final phase of life, efforts have to be focused on finding and maintaining a balance between the sense of integrity and the feeling of despair. When the sense of integrity is greater than the feeling of despair, the psychosocial strength that Erikson terms wisdom can be developed (Erikson 1997). Wisdom does not mean that a severely ill and dying person is free of conflicts and difficulties but that in spite of these, she is able to maintain her integrity and interest in life. The Eriksons are of the opinion that it is possible to become reconciled with one's bodily and mental losses. Furthermore, Joan Erikson argues that older people can in some cases attain *gerotranscendence*, referring to a definition provided by the Swedish researcher Lars Tornstam: 'In simple terms gerotranscendence means a change in the meta perspective, from a material and rational to a more cosmic and transcendent view, usually accompanied by enhanced satisfaction with life'. This corresponds to the state described by nursing researchers as *peace of mind* (Nyström & Andersson-Segesten 1990). Thus, according to the Eriksons' theory, identity development is possible throughout life, and this is supported by research and the thanatological literature. The psychiatrist and thanatologist Avery D. Weisman and his co-workers were among the first to establish that, from the patient's perspective, an appropriate death entailed more than merely being kept alive. Weisman coined the term 'significant survival' to denote that a person who is close to death retains a certain measure of quality of life and the concept of a purposeful death also includes personal development. A study of severely ill and dying patients provided concrete examples of both these concepts, where events were described that had involved a deepening or broadening of identity. The identity could even be extended close to death. One such example is Ann's experience of having become a grandmother a few months before her death. During conversations with her a couple of weeks before she died, she mentioned this fact several times. When asked if it made dying more difficult, she answered:

> It certainly makes it more difficult, but I've become accustomed to it and even accepted it. I've had time to say goodbye and sort things out. It's a big consolation that I'm a grandma and my son a dad and that I have a small grandchild. You can have that life meaning even close to death. And it may sound strange but I think that having a grandchild will make it easier for me to die. I can have an inner dialogue with him right up to the moment of death or for as long as I'm lucid. I think that will help me. It's a consolation that my grandchild will hear stories about me when I'm gone. In that way I will still be around. Now that I'm close to death, I'll die with a more positive picture of myself, more so than if I had died a few months ago. Then I would have died a poorer person (Ternestedt 2005).

It was reported that she retained her identity and a sense of dignity to the very end. As we cannot be certain about what Ann herself experienced in the final hours and minutes of her life, it is impossible to establish whether or not her death was dignified from her own perspective. She died with a positive feeling about life, and there is reason to believe that her dying and death were in line with her values. However, it is also important not to romanticise her experiences and death. Death can also be fraught with mental suffering. Research that focuses on the final phase of life has demonstrated that many dying people fluctuate between different feelings (James et al. 2007), for example hope and despair, as well as between the will to live and the wish to die (Qvarnström 1978). It is reasonable to assume that this was also the case with Ann. However, she appears to have maintained a feeling of integrity (see Erikson 1997), as she described how her identity was improved by the fact that she became a grandmother a few months before her death. Another person might have experienced this event in a different way. The birth of a grandchild could also pose a threat to one's identity, because of the sorrow and frustration involved in knowing that one will not live to see the child grow up. Ann's account highlights the fact that she had a social network that strengthened her perception of identity, an advantage that not everyone enjoys. Feelings of alienation and exclusion can threaten one's identity in the same way as not having access to the same care as others.

7.5   Threats to identity close to death

It is important not to romanticise death and dying or to moralise about the different ways in which people are perceived to cope with their end-of-life phase. Many factors can challenge a person's perception of her life, such as deterioration in bodily and mental functions (Lawton 2000). Joan Erikson (1997) described her own experiences following her husband's death as well as those of others in the end-of-life phase, and how losses and an increasing dependence on others challenge previously successful solutions to a crisis. In her experience, the development of wisdom was jeopardised by mistrust, shame, guilt, inferiority, confused identity, isolation, stagnation and despair. There is a risk that a severely ill or very old person in need of help will develop aversion and contempt instead of integrity and wisdom. However, in Joan Erikson's opinion, it is possible to become reconciled with one's bodily and mental losses. The way in which older people perceive themselves and their identity is considered highly dependent on the approach to them by society and people around them (Erikson 1997). Although David and Ann perceived meaningfulness close to death, their identity was at times threatened. Nevertheless, they succeeded in balancing these threats in a way that was beneficial to them. One likely explanation is their personalities as well as their previous strategies for coping with various crises. Weisman & Kastenbaum (1968) hold that dying people often use the same coping strategies at their life's end as they did in their previous life. Another important factor in David's and Ann's cases was that they had a supportive social network, which strengthened their sense of belonging. They chose to remain in their own home for as long as they were able, after which they opted to die in forms of care where specialist palliative care competence was available. Furthermore, they were lucky in that they had the opportunity to choose the form of care themselves. Care in the home is considered by many to be an intervention that promotes meaning in everyday life as well as identity and dignity. Several studies report that care in the home also strengthens feelings of independence and participation, making it easier to have control over one's own existence and be oneself as well as to maintain and develop relationships with others. However, not everyone experiences care in the home in a positive way, as it can pose a threat to a person's identity, for example when they are no longer able to take care of the home in the same way as previously or when the home is no longer safe from a medical or nursing perspective.

Many other factors can, of course, have a bearing on whether a person feels at ease in their own home or feels like a stranger there, which means that the person's identity is clearly threatened (Lawton 2000). The latter was the case with Diana, who was around 65 years old and had an advanced form of cancer. She had unwillingly had to retire on grounds of ill-health a couple of years previously. She had enjoyed her work, which formed a major part of her identity. She was married and had two adult children, with whom she had little contact. When her strength declined and she could no longer manage to leave her home without assistance, she experienced a great deterioration in her quality of life. She perceived that life had lost meaning. Diana described herself as being shut out from everything. Her home became a prison, making her more and more passive. Diana said: 'When you are ill and not so fit and alert it is easy to lose interest in things and to keep your dressing-gown on all day. I feel self-pity ... and I'm not alert in the evening if I didn't get up in the morning'. She stated that she had nothing but her disease and medication to talk to her husband about when he came home in the evening. She felt boring, ugly and ashamed at her lack of energy. She also found that her friends withdrew, which increased her feeling that she no longer had anything to contribute. Her previous positive self-image was not confirmed and she experienced that her value as a human being had been reduced. Her own explanation of why others withdrew was that her disease frightened them. She personified death, and her presence reminded others that death would eventually affect them too. Diana perceived herself to be both socially and existentially alone. She lived in a bubble and perceived herself as socially dead. Her identity was diminished. She was saved from these negative feelings when she was offered the opportunity to take part in day-care activities a couple of days each week. The transport service brought her to the day-care centre, where her life took on a new meaning. She had the opportunity to share experiences with others in a similar situation and was stimulated by various study visits. She found that her relationship with her husband improved, as she had something to talk about and could contribute, which meant that she once again experienced a sense of meaning and a sense that life was worth living. Her self-image and identity were strengthened.

The greatest threat to identity and dignity was described by nursing home residents. We have followed older people over time in several projects in order to study what they perceive to be a valuable life and a dignified death. In one study, 12 older individuals were followed over a period of 18 months (Franklin et al. 2006). Dwyer (2008) described both the threats to dignity experienced by older people and those perceived by staff as threatening their own self-respect when they were unable to provide the level of care they deemed appropriate and that was expected of them. The staff reported perceiving a wide gap between the ideals expressed at the societal level and the means at their disposal for realising them in their daily work. They stated that the organisation did not allow individualised care, in which conversation and time together were natural components of daily life. They also considered that the dignity of the older people was threatened and gave expression to what Glasberg et al. (2007) have termed 'conscience stress'. They also reported that they had no opportunity to achieve the good things they wanted to do.

The older people in Dwyer's study described a sense of alienation due to not feeling at home in the nursing home, despite the fact that it provided them with security, as they were dependent on others for assistance. In addition, they felt alienated in relation to their own body. One bodily function after another failed, and the day when they could no longer control their urine and faeces meant a clear violation of their identity and dignity. Dwyer et al. (2008) have described how the older people tried to create meaning in their life by conducting an inner dialogue with themselves, when they recalled pleasant memories that had meant a great deal to them. In another study Mary, who was 98 years old, physically disabled and blind, considered that she did not gain much benefit from the other residents. She was one of the most alert residents and found it difficult to conduct a conversation at the dinner table, as most of the older people there were very hard of hearing. However, Mary created meaning in her everyday life by conducting an inner dialogue. She thought about the times when she was the owner of a small shop and in her mind she continued to sell newspapers and other items. She could quickly calculate the total cost of the items. She was proud of her preserved cognitive ability and retained her zest for life (Ternestedt & Franklin 2006), which strengthened her self-image and sense of identity. For Sara, who was almost 100 years old, the situation was different. She was completely bedridden and very much dependent on the staff. Despite having had exciting periods in her life, thinking about it did not afford her any pleasure. She found life meaningless and was unable to obtain solace from the staff members' approach to her. She was very dissatisfied and even expressed a loathing of herself and others. She longed for only one thing and that was to die. From the dying person's perspective, death can come too early, at the right point in time or too late. In Sara's case, her view was that death came too late.

Common to David, Ann, Diana, Mary and Sara was that disease/ageing was experienced as a threat to their identity, which Nordenfelt has termed *dignity of identity* (see Chapter 2). The conduct of staff members was described as being critical with regard to whether or not the older persons considered that their dignity had been preserved. In some cases, staff members' behaviour was compensatory, i.e. it strengthened the sense of meaningfulness in everyday life as well as the older person's self-image. Many of the older people were of the opinion that staff did their best, and that the deficiencies lay in the way the work was organised and inadequate staff support. The lack of resources that characterised the nursing homes was seen as a signal at the societal level that older people do not have the same worth as others and are therefore marginalised. This view largely corresponds to the description of older persons' situation in the WHO report mentioned above (WHO 2004a).

7.6 Identity-promoting care

The above examples more or less clearly demonstrate the way in which the interplay between individuals and their surroundings can both promote and threaten the dying person's identity and experience of dignity. Furthermore, the ageing process and the disease itself often constitute a threat to identity and dignity. An implicit finding was the importance of the caring culture in which older and dying people live being characterised by rituals built on a dynamic interplay between staff and client. There is a risk

159

of this interplay stagnating and becoming stereotyped for various reasons, which can be compared to what Erikson (1997) described as 'ritualism'. The caring culture described by the elderly people can be said to be strongly characterised by such ritualism.

For several years, the work of our research group has focused on the development of a thought model that is based on a caring perspective aimed at promoting the opportunities for seriously ill and dying patients to experience a good and dignified death. In this context, dignity has been defined as being allowed to be the person one is until death. This means that caring should promote the possibilities of individuals living their last days in accordance with their life philosophy and lifestyle (provided that this is what they want). The patient's or older person's right of self-determination is therefore central in the design of care. Our thought model takes its ontological standpoint from a perspective on humanity which embraces the view that an individual is capable of development throughout life, within the limits set by disease and ageing. This is in line with the Erikson's (1997) theory about individual identity and psychosocial development from birth until death. Central to their theory is that soma, psyche and ethos constitute a whole, which is also the case in the thought framework outlined below. This framework is well supported by research in the area of dying and death. It can also be said to fulfil the needs of a dying person, irrespective of whether their values correspond to traditional, modern or postmodern death, or a combination of the three.

The initial inspiration for the development of the thought model was the research of the thanatologist Avery D. Weisman. In his early writings he stressed that, from the patient's perspective, a good and dignified death (he used the term 'appropriate death') meant more than being kept alive. The care should promote the person's quality of life, a goal similar to that of hospice philosophy and palliative care. Weisman repeatedly emphasised that the only person who can be the judge of what dignity means to him is the dying person himself, which calls for an individualisation of care. Weisman & Kastenbaum (1968) also described a method that aims to learn, from every person's dying and death, knowledge that could be utilised in the encounter with the next person. This method was developed during a period when autopsies were commonly used to establish the cause of death. Weisman, who wished to learn more about the deceased person's psychosocial life and how they had lived, thought or felt in relation to their own death, called his method 'psychological autopsy'. The method involved gathering the care team members together shortly after a person's death and focusing on a number of questions from a patient perspective. This method had previously been used within nursing research (Andersson-Segesten 1989). Weisman focused on the following questions: (1) Did the patient have adequate medical care and relief from pain toward the end of life? (2) How completely did the patient manage his or her life up until the time of death? (3) To what degree did the patient maintain rewarding or significant relationships during the terminal period? (4) Did the patient die with a decent self-image and a feeling of personal significance? (5) Were there signs of conflict resolution? (6) Was there personal consent to die?

These six questions were translated into Swedish (Rinell Hermansson 1990) and six keywords formulated, all beginning with the letter S (Hermansson & Ternestedt 2000). These six S keywords are *symptom control, self-determination, social relationships, self-image, synthesis* and *surrender*. The questions and keywords were then adapted by means of concept derivation to a nursing context, in which the model was tested (Ternestedt

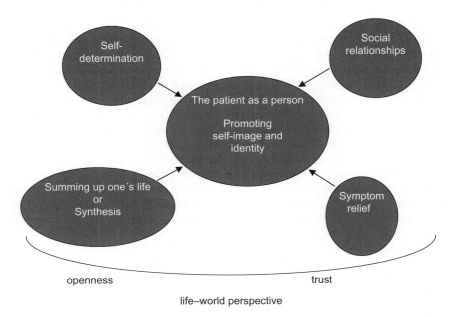

Figure 7.1 Person-centred and identity-promoting care.

et al. 2002). Today, this thought model, called the *six S keywords*, is used in several palliative care units in Sweden.

We began our development work on the model in conjunction with the establishment of a hospice at a university hospital in Sweden, where we were assigned to evaluate the activities. We have followed hospice activities since that time (Andershed & Ternestedt 1997; Rinell Hermansson & Ternestedt 2000; Sahlberg Blom 2001; Källström Karlsson et al. 2006, 2008). The criteria that we developed (the six S keywords) cover aspects of the patient's physical, psychological, social and spiritual/existential needs and can also be regarded as an operationalisation of the WHO definition of palliative care. The relations between five of the six S's are illustrated in Figure 7.1, which has been specially adapted to care planning.

Figure 7.1 illustrates the fact that it is the individual who is the obvious point of departure in care planning. The intention is that the patient and, when the patient so wishes, the next of kin, should play an active role in the planning of the care. The six S keywords can be used to facilitate discussions aimed at getting to know the patient and, not least, at understanding how the patient and the family members think and feel in relation to the disease. The challenge for the nurse is thereby to confirm the patient/ older person and listen to their narrative without the use of coercion or manipulation. Repeated daily conversations are necessary in order to obtain sufficient information. The purpose of the six S keywords is to support the person's possibilities of preserving as much as possible of their identity. However, this requires knowledge on the part of carers that the S keywords can have a different loading for different people. What is the future scenario envisaged by the various family members? How do they think, feel and act? And how does the sick person wish to spend their final period of life together with their next of kin (if any)? How can the care promote the dying person's possibilities of retaining a self-image that is as positive as possible? As Figure 7.1 illustrates, the core of the thought model is the S that indicates self-image, which concerns who the patient or the elderly person describes themself to be. The meaning of self-image is close to the term 'dignity of identity' (Nordenfelt 2004; Nordenfelt, this volume, Chapter 2).

Four of the six S keywords – self-determination, social relationships, symptom control and summing up/synthesis – are criteria that concern a person's self-image, identity and dignity. The criterion of surrender concerns the dying person's acceptance or reconciliation with the fact that death is close. It is not unusual for someone approaching the end of life to wish to complete something before dying, or finalise a project or relationship that means a great deal to them. This can, for example, apply to practical matters.

The six S keywords or criteria of good and dignified end-of-life care do not constitute a norm that should be forced on someone or to which the dying process should be adapted. The aim of the model is quite the opposite. It should promote the dying person's chances of dying in the manner of their own choice, in accord with their values and outlook on life. The six S keywords are intended to guide carers in the identification of social, psychological, spiritual/existential and physical needs, including the need for symptom relief and good bodily care. Each person's death is unique, although there are common features. Individual differences mean that a dying person requires individualised support and care. Some people only want the health professionals to help them with the relief of physical symptoms, while their other needs are satisfied elsewhere. Others have a strong need to talk about their life over and over again to someone who listens actively and shows respect for their narrative. Such a narrative can be of vital importance for a person's experience of identity. Accordingly, it is important to be aware that the six S keywords have a different loading for different people and can even vary for the same person according to circumstances. Although a person may be unwilling to talk about their life on one occasion, that does not preclude the possibility that they may want to do so another day. It is therefore important for health-care staff to update their information about the care plan on a regular basis, as needs can change at the end of life in the same way as they do during life. The content of the six S keywords agrees with the findings of other studies in this area and can therefore be considered knowledge-based. In addition, the thought model is the result of many years of research. A brief description of examples of question areas that concretise the content of the six S keywords is given in Box 7.1.

In this chapter examples of the six S keywords have been presented as a thought model applicable to care planning. The model can equally be used for the documentation and evaluation of palliative care (Ternestedt 1998; Rinell Hermansson & Ternestedt 2000; Ternestedt et al. 2002; Ternestedt 2007). Results from studies in which the model was used after a person's death to evaluate the care provided and identify potential areas for improvement (what we call retrospective analysis) reveal that, in general, health-care professionals know very little about their elderly clients, what their life was like before their illness and what was important to them (Andersson-Segesten 1989;

Box 7.1 Examples of the content of the six S keywords and supporting questions in palliative care planning

---

Self-image: The basis of each individual's self-description; obtain a picture of who the person is and what is of central importance in their life *(outlook on life and lifestyle)*
  Examples of supporting questions: Who are the people? What has been and is important to them? How do they experience their illness and situation? How can the care be designed so as to promote each individual's self-image? (the need to be a whole person, body and mind intertwined).

Self-determination: Based on each individual's needs and wishes, support the person so that they are involved in the care as much as possible *(psychological needs)*
  Examples of supporting questions: How dependent is the patient and how do they react to dependency? How can the person be supported in their struggle to achieve autonomy and the best possible quality of life? How can the care be designed so as to promote each individual's self-determination?

Social relationships: The basis of each individual's needs and wishes; support the person in maintaining or developing important social relationships and meeting relatives and friends in the way they wish *(social needs)*
  Examples of supporting questions: Which relationships are important to the person? How does the person want to balance a possible need for solitude with the need for belonging? How can the care be designed so as to meet each individual's social needs?

Symptom control: Alleviate symptoms in an optimal way according to each individual's needs and wishes *(physical and bodily needs)*
  Examples of supporting questions: What kind of symptoms does the person have? How can these symptoms be controlled? How can alternative therapy be employed? How can the care be designed so as to meet each individual's needs and wishes in the area of symptom relief?

Synthesis: The basis of each individual's needs and wishes; promote possibilities of creating and recognising continuity and meaning in the life they have lived as well as in the present *(spiritual/existential needs)*
  Examples of supporting questions: How does the person view death and the meaning of life? Does the person have a need to talk about their life? If so, how is this need met? How can the care be designed so as to meet each individual's spiritual and existential needs in accordance with their wishes?

Surrender: The basis of each individual's needs and wishes; promote possibilities of accepting or reconciling themself with the fact that death is imminent.
  Examples of supporting questions: How does the person react to being told that death is imminent? How are they given consolation? How can the care be designed so as to support the individual in their effort to reach closure in accordance with their own wishes?

Dwyer 2008). These studies, carried out at an interval of approximately 10 years, revealed that the staff had limited knowledge of what older people thought and felt in relation to their own death. Conversations about death were rare and the staff received no guidance or support.

It may be questioned whether the framework of the six S keywords is applicable in cases where a person is no longer capable of communicating their wishes because of extreme exhaustion, unconsciousness or advanced dementia, for example. However, it is reasonable to assume that even in such cases the six criteria can serve as guidance. Nevertheless, more research is required in this area.

7.7 Conclusion and reflections

Dying is a unique experience; only the dying person knows what constitutes a dignified death for them and is capable of deciding how they want to live their final days with the restrictions imposed by the illness, providing the condition has not impaired their cognitive faculties. Each individual is unique and has different values and aims in life, which implies that a good death can take many different forms. Good palliative care is responsive to patients' needs, which presupposes that it is planned in a dialogue with the patient and the next of kin. This requires carers who are knowledgeable, sensitive and flexible and who have a good sense of judgement.

The account of David shows a person who was privileged in many respects. He had his own resources, including those in his social environment. The same can be said of Ann. However, that was not the reason for presenting the accounts of David and Ann. Rather, the aim was to demonstrate the complexity of death and the need for care that is flexible and honest in order to help seriously ill or dying patients to live their last days as comfortably as possible and in accordance with their own lifestyle and outlook on life. For both David and Ann, their home played a major role. David refused home care in the final phase of his life, as he felt more secure and could be himself to a greater degree in a palliative care unit, where he felt comfortable. Ann also died in a palliative care unit, but for medical reasons. Her wish was to die in her own home surrounded by familiar objects and her family, but that did not happen.

For most people, the home has a positive connotation and it has been described as an extension of one's personal identity. Several studies reveal, either implicitly or explicitly, that home care can promote a person's identity. However, the home may also have negative connotations; it may, for example, be associated with abuse or isolation, thus posing a threat to a person's identity and dignity. A nursing home that is experienced as home promotes identity and dignity, but one in which the person does not feel at home constitutes a threat to identity. The meaning of the concept 'home' can and should be problematised. In contemporary society, the definition of 'home' is not obvious. Like many other Western countries, Sweden is characterised by a high degree of mobility. It is common for people to work in one location and to live in another, or to have two homes, one of which functions as the permanent family home and the other as a base for work. A person may feel equally at home in both dwellings. Today, many children whose parents are divorced grow up with two homes. It is not unusual for children to live for one week with their mother and the next week with their father, provided that the parents live fairly close to each other. It is reasonable to assume that this situation can lead to a change in the significance of home (and locality) to one's identity.

This chapter represents an attempt to demonstrate that the self and one's identity can continue to develop throughout life, i.e. even including the final phase. Erikson & Erikson (1997) have shown that development is possible even when the functioning of vital bodily organs begins to fail. This perspective is supported by the studies of the thanatologist Avery D. Weisman on dying and death in different care settings, as well as by some empirical studies with the focus on the self or identity. To date, relatively few studies have investigated the development of identity in the dying process. However, there are studies that describe different nursing methods that promote identity and dignity (Chochinov et al. 2002; Chochinov 2006), of which the six S keywords are an example. The point of departure of the six S keywords is the older person's need, outlook on life and lifestyle. The framework is intended to facilitate the promotion of a dying person's possibility of being the person they are until death (identity-promoting care) and can also be used for the documentation and evaluation of palliative care.

In addition, it is pointed out in this chapter that there is a need for further development to ensure that the aims of palliative care can be achieved within various care settings, to enable as many people as possible to experience a dignified end of life. This is another area that requires further research.

The three perspectives on death – traditional, modern and postmodern – will hopefully help us to be open, both with ourselves and with others. We live in a multicultural society that embraces many different views on what constitutes a good life and a good death. The era in which we live is also characterised by a strong body culture, and the emphasis on independence can often undermine our sense of natural human dependence. It cannot be taken for granted that autonomy is a major priority at the end of life, and this requires additional research. The three perspectives on death mentioned above could broaden our frame of reference in encounters with individuals who have, for example, a different cultural background. They might even help us to better understand what constitutes a dignified death for a person, who, for various reasons, is unable to communicate their wishes. In such cases, care with dignity is based on available knowledge concerning how a person previously lived their life and what was important to them. This knowledge can increase our chances of ensuring that an individual has as dignified a death as possible.

References

Andershed, B. & Ternestedt, B.-M. (1997) Patterns of care for patients with cancer before and after the establishment of a hospice ward. *Scandinavian Journal of Caring Sciences*, **11**, 42–50.

Andersson-Segesten, K. (1989) The last period of life of the very old. A pilot study evaluating the psychological autopsy method. *Scandinavian Journal of Caring Sciences*, **3**, 177–181.

Bauman, Z. (1992) *Mortality, Immortality and Other Life Strategies*. Stanford University Press, Stanford, CA.

Callahan, D. (1993) Pursuing a peaceful death. *Hastings Center Report*, **23**, July–August, 22–28.

Chochinov, H.M. (2006) Dying, dignity, and new horizons in palliative end-of-life care. *CA: A Cancer Journal for Clinicians*, **56**, 84–103.

Chochinov, H.M., Hack, T.M., McClement, S., Kristjanson, L. & Harlos, M. (2002) Dignity in the terminally ill: a developing empirical model. *Social Science and Medicine*, **54**, 433–443.

Clark, D. (2007/2008) End-of-life care around the world: achievements to date and challenges remaining. *Omega*, **56**, 101–110.

Connor, S.R. (2007/2008) Development of hospice and palliative care in the United States. *Omega*, **56**, 89–99.

Dwyer, L.L. (2008) Dignity in the End of Life Care. What Does it Mean to Older People and Staff in Nursing Homes? PhD thesis, Örebro University.

Dwyer, L.L., Nordenfelt, L. & Ternestedt, B.-M. (2008) Three nursing home residents speak about meaning at the end of life. *Nursing Ethics*, **15**, 88–100.

Erikson, E.H. (1997) *The Life Cycle Completed*. Extended version with new chapters on the ninth stage of development by Joan M Erikson. Norton, New York.

Franklin, L.L., Nordenfelt, L. & Ternestedt, B.-M. (2006) Views on dignity of elderly nursing home residents. *Nursing Ethics*, **13**, 130–146.

Fryback, P.B. (1993) Health for people with a terminal diagnosis. *Nursing Science Quarterly*, **6**, 147–159.

Glasberg, A.L., Erikson, S. & Norberg, A. (2007) Burnout and 'stress of conscience' among healthcare personnel. *Journal of Advanced Nursing*, **57**, 392–403.

Goodridge, D., Bond, J.B. Jr., Cameron, C. and McKean, E. (2005) End-of-life care in a nursing home: a study of family, nurse and healthcare aide perspectives. *International Journal of Palliative Nursing*, **11**, 226–232.

Hermansson, A.R. & Ternestedt, B.-M. (2000) What do we know about the dying patient? Awareness as a means to improve palliative care. *Medicine and Law*, **19**, 335–344.

Jakobsson, E., Johnsson, T., Persson, L.O. & Gaston-Johansson, F. (2006) End-of-life in a Swedish population: demographics, social conditions and characteristics of places of death. *Scandinavian Journal of Caring Science*, **20**, 10–17.

James, I., Andershed, B. & Ternestedt, B.-M. (2007) A family's beliefs about cancer, dying and death in the end of life. *Journal of Family Nursing*, **13**, 226–252.

Källström Karlsson, I.L., Ehnfors, M. & Ternestedt, B.-M. (2006) Patient characteristics of women and men cared for during the first 10 years at an inpatient hospice ward in Sweden. *Scandinavian Journal of Caring Sciences*, **20**, 113–121.

Källström Karlsson, I.L., Ehnfors, M. & Ternestedt, B.-M. (2008) Five nurses experiences of hospice care in a long term perspective. *Journal of Hospice and Palliative Nursing*, **10**, 224–232.

Lawton, J. (2000) *The Dying Process. Patients' Experiences of Palliative Care*. Routledge & Kegan Paul, London.

Lloyd, L. (2004) Mortality and morality; ageing and the ethics of care. *Ageing and Society*, **24**, 235–256.

McNamara, B., Waddell, C. & Colvin, M. (1995) The institutionalisation of the good death. *Social Science and Medicine*, **39**, 1501–1508.

Meier, D.E., Morrison, R.S. & Cassel, C.K.J. (1997) Improving palliative care. *Annals of Internal Medicine*, **127**, 225–230.

Nordenfelt, L. (2004) The varieties of dignity. *Health Care Analysis*, **12**, 69–81.

Nyström, A.M. & Andersson-Segesten, K. (1990) Peace of mind as an important aspect of old people's health. *Scandinavian Journal of Caring Sciences*, **4**, 55–62.

Payne, S.A., Langley-Evans, A. & Hillier, R. (1996) Perceptions of a good death: a comparative study of the views of hospice staff and patients. *Palliative Medicine*, **10**, 307–312.

Qvarnström, U. (1978) Patients' Reactions to Impending Death. A Clinical Study. PhD thesis, Stockholm University.

Rinell Hermansson, A. (1990) Det sista året. Omsorg och vård vid livets slut [The last year. Care at the end of life]. (In Swedish with a summary in English) PhD thesis, Uppsala University.

Russel, P. & Sander, R. (1998) Palliative care: promoting the concept of a healthy death. *British Journal of Nursing*, **7**, 256–261.

Sahlberg Blom, E. (2001) Autonomy, Dependency and Quality of Life. The Last Month of Life for 56 Cancer Patients. PhD thesis, Uppsala University.

Seymour, J., Witherspoon, R., Gott, M., Ross, J., Payne, S. & Owen, T. (2005) *End of Life Care: Promoting Comfort, Choice and Well Being for Older People*. Policy Press, Bristol.

Snyder, R.D. (1994) Changing of shift. A peaceful death. *Annals of Emergency Medicine*, **24**, 1195–1196.

Ternestedt, B.-M. (1998) *Livet Pågår! – Om vård av döende* [*Life goes on! – On the care of dying patients*]. Studentlitteratur, Lund.

Ternestedt, B.-M. (2005) Hjälp att leva livet ut [Help to live]. In: *Att få hjälp att dö – synsätt, erfarenheter, kritiska frågor* [*Obtaining assistance to die – perspectives, experiences and key issues*]. (eds C.-G. Westrin and T. Nilstun), pp. 73–88. Studentlitteratur, Lund.

Ternestedt, B.-M. (2007) Att få vara den man är i dödens närhet [To be allowed to be the person you are when close to death]. In: *Hemmets vårdetik: Om vård av äldre i livets slutskede* [*The care of older people at the end of life: The ethics of care in the home*]. (ed G. Silfverberg), pp. 147–163. Studentlitteratur, Lund. (In Swedish)

Ternestedt, B.-M. & Franklin, L.L. (2006) Ways of relating to death: views of older people resident in nursing homes. *International Journal of Palliative Nursing*, **12**, 334–340. (Erratum in *International Journal of Palliative Nursing*, 2006, **12**, 544.)

Ternestedt, B.-M., Andershed, B., Eriksson, M. & Johansson, I. (2002) A good death. Development of a nursing model of care. *Journal of Hospice and Palliative Nursing*, **4**, 153–160.

Twycross, R. (2007/2008) Looking back and looking forward. Patient care: past, present, and future. *Omega*, **56**, 7–19.

Vachon, M.L.S. (2001) The stress of professional caregivers. In: *Oxford Textbook of Palliative Medicine* (eds D. Doyle, G.W.C. Hanks, and N. MacDonald), pp. 919–929. Oxford University Press, Oxford.

Walter, T. (1994) *The Revival of Death*. Routledge & Kegan Paul, London.

Weisman, A.D. (1974) *The Realization of Death. A Guide for the Psychological Autopsy*. Jason Aronson, New York.

Weisman, A.D. & Kastenbaum, R. (1968) The psychological autopsy. A study of the terminal phase of life. *Community Mental Health Journal*, Monograph **4**. Behavioral Publications, New York.

Whitaker, A. (2004) Livets sista boning. Anhörigskap, åldrande och död på sjukhem [*The final home. Family ties, ageing and death in a nursing home*]. (In Swedish with a summary in English). PhD thesis, Stockholm University.

WHO (2004a) *Better Palliative Care for Older People*, World Health Organization, Copenhagen.

WHO (2004b) *Solid Facts: Palliative Care*. World Health Organization, Copenhagen.

8. *Dignity and the Dead*

Göran Lantz

Introduction

My point of departure for these reflections on the status of the dead and the dignity of the dead is my own experience. I was present when my father, my mother and my only brother died. None of these deaths took place in a hospital setting. I have attended post-mortem examinations, and I have lectured to medical students in connection with their first encounter with such examinations. I have interviewed doctors, priests, undertakers, public transporters of dead bodies and other professionals who deal with the dead. The purpose of my interviews has not been to survey the whole problematic field or to attempt a representative mapping of attitudes or opinions, but rather to search for wise and well-informed ideas to aid my own reflections.

8.1   The view of the dead person

The view of the dead person is a question of the actual seeing of the body from a specific perspective in a specific situation. The perspective of the mourning relative and the perspective of a pathologist differ widely. And so do the perspectives of all the other people (lay or professional) who have to deal with the dead. But the view of the dead person may also stand for what I would like to call the phenomenology of the dead. Just as we talk of anthropology we may talk of a *thananthropology* of the dead, which is the view of the dead in a philosophical sense. The view of the dead person in this sense is obviously a social construct, but it is still a deeply rooted and stable view and very difficult to change. I take it that thananthropology is culturally determined and may change over time and between cultures. This chapter of course reflects my own position as a Christian Swedish academic, but I think it might be relevant for a 'Western' view in general. I will try to avoid (or at least, when relevant, account for) a specific religious or Christian outlook.

The mere physical act of seeing is invariably connected with a specific interpretation of the object that is seen. Seeing without interpretation or understanding is extremely exceptional. Only a deeply aphasic person can 'see' something in this sense.

The word 'see' is often used in a very wide sense. The expression 'I see' is synonymous with 'I understand'. St Augustine remarks that sight is the most inclusive sensation. Consequently, for him *visio Dei*, seeing God, means not actually looking at God, but experiencing God in a comprehensive sense (the highest experience of God).

Seeing can be delusional. The sight of something can clearly be misinterpreted. When I saw my brother in hospital shortly after his death I saw his chest moving. This was obviously an illusion caused by my normal expectation that a person breathes and that their chest rises. It illustrates the fact that there is a remarkable psychological delay in our experience of the person as dead. To take another example from my own experience: sitting at my father's deathbed, I did not at one moment see my father alive and then at the moment immediately after his death see a corpse, a mere thing. I first saw my father as living and then saw my father as dead, my dead father.

This delay is a psychological phenomenon. But it is also a fact that death is something gradual. Different organs will die at different moments since they are dependent on oxygen to varying degrees. Socially, there is also delay in our experience of the dead. The dead person is normally felt to be 'alive' for the relatives for a long time, let's say until the moment of farewell, perhaps until the funeral. On the other hand, a person might be thought of as dead long before their biological death (for instance, during a long period of deep dementia or coma).

The view of the dead person can be more or less reductionist and more or less holistic. One extreme is, as already said, the totally aphasic view, the seeing of a mere thing. Another extreme could be the view from the pathologist's angle. But this is not an example of a totally reductionist view. Even for the pathologist the corpse is seen as a human body and not as a mere thing.

The view of the person as dead is more holistic in so far as it includes the grasp of a fuller identity of that person. What, then, is the identity of a person, alive or dead? I am my body, but I am also my memory. In my view the identity in the latter sense is essential. We can distinguish between what William James called the 'I' and the 'Me'. The 'I' is the abstract subject of all of my sensations and experiences. It can be compared with Immanuel Kant's concept of the transcendental ego. In a modern version presented by the Swedish philosopher Erik Ryding it can be described as the 'I zero', the abstract focal point of sensations. It is an empty ego, whereas the 'Me' is the ego filled with a content of characteristics of all kinds. It contains, so to speak, the full picture of the person.

In my view the 'Me' in this sense is identical with a person's life story. Since we understand ourselves in terms of a story, we are, as Alasdair McIntyre, puts it, 'story-telling animals'. That is to say, we organise our identity not only in terms of physical causal explanations but also and above all in terms of intentional explanations, since human action needs intentional explanations (Nordenfelt 2000, pp. 29–46; von Wright 2004, pp. 1–33). Normally we tell other people who we are not in physiological but in narrative terms. Quite simply, I am my life story (Lantz 1997, pp. 64–66).

The idea of the life story as an essential aspect of a person's identity, the narrative aspect, has many implications for care. Health care is not only about caring for bodies but also about caring for life stories. Privacy, for instance, is about respect for and cultivation of the identity of people in terms of respect for their life stories.

Telling the story of a person entails an aspect of power. It implies defining the identity of the person. We can distinguish between first-person telling and second- and third-person telling.

- *First-person telling* means the person's own narrative. When I tell my life story, or part of it, I define myself, who I am. From my own perspective my story is a product not only of what I have done and experienced, but also a product of how I have understood and interpreted what has happened to me. That is to say, my narrative identity can be more or less authentic. It can be misunderstood and misinterpreted. I can have a wishful identity or a more realistic story of myself. I exercise power when telling about myself. Ideally a person tells her identity in terms of a true, authentic, story, with both self-criticism and pride. She has taken control of her identity.
- *Second-person telling* is the special case when we ascribe a narrative identity to each other in a dialogue.
- *Third-person telling* is when someone from an outsider's perspective tells who another person is. This is also an exercise of power, not least because such third-person telling might include defining the person's character, her vices and virtues. But the very telling in itself, even a morally neutral telling, is exercising power as far as the third person defines another person. Such third-person telling is inevitable in daily life as well as in a doctor–patient relationship. To use this power over people need not be wrong or offensive.

The power of telling might be an act of healing or an act of reverence, both very positive contributions to a person's identity. Instances of healing are when the psychologist or psychiatrist tries to reconstruct the identity of her patient. The identity of a psychotic patient can be understood as a life story that is fragmented and unintelligible. The role of the health professional is then to make the narrative identity of the patient whole and unbroken, in short to make it *integer*. Nevertheless, this constitutes an exercise of power, albeit a positive power. The narration in itself is an act of power, and it is obvious that the life story of a person can be treated with reverence and piety as well as with disrespect or contempt.

The end of a life story is of special significance. At the moment of a person's death we have, so to speak, the result of her life. Words uttered just before death might be of great importance and weight. They cannot be changed. They remain as the last impression of the dead person. This impression colours as it were the whole story of the person. There is a whole genre of stories about what happened and what was said in the last moments of life. The end of life is an important part of the whole life. Sometimes it is integrated into the life story and the identity of the person in a remarkable way. That is the case with the death of Jesus or of Socrates.

> Death does not always mark the boundary of a person's life as an end that stands outside it; sometimes it is a part of that life, continuing its narrative story in some significant way (Nozick 1990, p. 23).

Moreover, a person's last wish demands respect and obedience both morally and in certain circumstances legally. At the end of life we have access to the complete life story. We think we can sum up the person's deeds and character, but this is only partly true. Imagine a person who in his life was kind, loving and pious. His life was characterised by just these virtues, and this is true at the moment of his death. But a couple of days after his death it is revealed that he had a child out of wedlock which he had not dared to tell his family about. Now, some time after his death his character might be summed up not only as kind, loving and pious, but also as cowardly and untruthful. His narrative identity can be altered long after his death. There is a proverb in the Icelandic *Hávamál* that says, 'Beasts die, kinsmen die, you yourself die; one thing I know that never dies, and that is the judgement of the dead man'.

Let me sum up: The human person has her identity in a *diachronic* perspective, and this perspective has both a retrospective and a prospective aspect. From the retrospective point of view her identity is her life story. From the prospective point of view her identity is her life plan, i.e. her plans and expectations with regard to her future life.

But the person has also her identity in a *synchronic* perspective. She is the person she is as part of a social context. As Charles Taylor put it, 'What we are as human beings we are only in a cultural community' (Taylor 1985, pp. 206–207). One could also say that the individual life story is part of a greater story, including not only the story of the individual but also the story of family and nation. Ultimately we are part of the history of mankind. The 17th-century English poet John Donne, gives fine expression to this thought in a well-known passage:

> Here the bells can scarcely solemnise the funeral of any person, but that I knew him, or knew that he was my neighbour. We dwelt in houses near to one another before, but now he is gone into that house into which I must follow him ... No man is an island, entire of itself; every man is a piece of the continent, a part of the mainland. If a clod be washed away by the sea, Europe is the less, as well as if a promontory were, as well as if a manor of thy friends or of thine own were. Any man's death diminishes me, because I am involved in mankind. And therefore never send to know for whom the bell tolls. It tolls for thee.

The dead person is no longer the subject of her life story, although she is still the main figure of this life story. She is no longer a transcendental ego, or an 'I' in James's sense. But the life story is still there, and she is still the main character of this story. Her narrative identity remains. The life story is part of other life stories and survives in those stories. So, diachronically (retrospectively but not prospectively) and synchronically the identity of the dead person is still there.

Is there a specific Christian thananthropology? I think so, just as there is a specific Christian anthropology, or rather several forms of Christian anthropology. I take it that a mainstream Christian anthropology includes the idea that God created Man in His image and that every individual person is the object of His love and care. This makes the individual enormously important and valuable in a Christian view. Man has eternal life. Therefore God's care for him does not stop at the moment of death. Thus a Christian embraces the idea that the dead person is also important and valuable. A similar idea holds true for other religious views of the dead, for instance the Jewish or Muslim. In Christian theology there has been a debate as to whether the dead will arise as a new creation or their souls will survive until the Day of Judgement. It has been maintained that the latter view is less firmly established in biblical thought. But this need not affect the idea of the high esteem of the dead in Christian thought. Admittedly the introduction of cremation as a form of funeral caused some resistance among Christian churches, but today cremation is accepted by most churches and is not seen as disrespectful towards the deceased. It does not contradict the idea of humanity, alive or dead, as part of God's plan for salvation. The individual life story is, as already said, part of the story of salvation. I will return to further religious aspects below.

8.2   The dead as persons

The concept of a person is notoriously difficult. Personhood includes not only belonging to the human race, but normally also having certain characteristics such as rationality, self-consciousness and the capability of moral reasoning. It is usually thought to give rise to rights and duties. That is to say, personhood, the concept of a person, belongs to a moral discourse. 'The concept of a person, unlike that of a human being, which is simply a biological category, is in part at least a moral concept' (Brecher 2002).

We apply the concept of a person to people in order to assign to them (1) value or dignity, (2) rights and (3) duties and responsibility. In what sense, then, can the deceased human being be said to be a person? Since the dead person in the holistic view that I have advocated is still the main figure in her life story and since she is part of other people's life stories, I think it is fair to say that she is still a person. From the diachronic point of view (the retrospective but not the prospective) and from the synchronic point of view a person as dead carries a holistic, i.e. a narrative, identity. She is still a part of a moral context. As Brecher puts it, 'in some ways you do not cease to be a person after you are dead; and to the extent that you remain (if you do) part of a community, you remain a person, even though a dead person' (Brecher 2002, p. 115).

So much for the moral aspect of being a person. But the concept of a person is not only a moral but also a legal concept. Is a dead person a person in the legal sense? In jurisprudence the concept of a *legal person* is ascribed to companies, firms or foundations as well as to individuals. Consider the following sentences:

X is 75 years old.

X has sold a car.

X is obliged to pay the debt.

X has received a gift.

X moves from Sweden to Britain.

X accepts the agreement.

All these six statements can be made about a legal person, such as for instance a company, but they can also be made about a physical person. The legal person can act, can have intentions, can have interests, and can have obligations and rights. And so of course can a physical person. In one analysis of the concept of a legal person the concept is seen as fictive, as alluding to a fictitious entity. But a realistic interpretation makes such a presumption of a fictitious entity unnecessary. Statements about a legal person can be understood as statements about rights, duties, acts and so forth in respect of affairs of fact that involve rights and so on arising from acts performed by physical persons in their capacities as representing or constituting a legal person. In this view the legal person is real and its acts are real (Moritz 1970).

How far does the parallel between the concept of a legal person and a physical person apply to the deceased? It is obvious that the estate of a deceased person is a legal person. But the legal concept of such an estate is not identical with that of the dead person. It is likewise clear that the dead person cannot act and thus cannot be a legal subject. But it is also obvious that the dead person is a legal object in the sense of being protected by legal rights. The dead person can have rights in both the moral and the legal sense. I shall return to this later in the chapter.

8.3   Change and continuity

The moment of death is an absolute borderline between life and death. It is the most radical change conceivable for a human being. Birth and death constitute the framework of human life. But just as becoming a human being is a gradual process, so is death. The beginning of human life is a highly contested subject. From the moment of fertilisation up to the delivery, different borderlines have been drawn for the start of personal life with all its moral and legal consequences. Death, as previously stated, is a gradual process. On the cellular level it might be quite difficult to observe the difference between material taken from living and dead bodies. Different parts of the body die at different times. Traditionally, the moment of death has been associated with the ceasing of respiration and/or the extinction of heart activity. New medical insights and possibilities have led to a concept of death related to the irrevocable cessation of the coordinating activities of the brain.

As I have already observed, the psychological experience of witnessing death may vary widely. On the one hand there is the impression of a person as dead long before the moment of actual death (for instance, of the irreversibly comatose or demented person). On the other hand the dead person may appear as alive and present well after this moment.

From the legal point of view, death also represents a radical change. Generally it is the change from a legal status comprising all the rights and duties of a living person to the legal status of a dead person with the specific rights that involves. More specifically, it is an important change transferring rules of inheritance.

So much for the change. But there is also a remarkable continuity between the living person and the dead person. As I said earlier, death is not the momentary transition from a person to a mere thing. First you experience your living father and after his death you experience your father, although he is dead; i.e. he is your dead father.

The *corporeal continuity* is obvious. The visual impression of the living and the newly dead is almost the same. A person who is dead in the technical sense of being without the coordinating activity of the brain but attached to a ventilator, a so-called brain-dead person, looks quite the same and, at least for the layman without access to highly sophisticated means of examination, can hardly be distinguished from a living person. (More about this below.)

Just as there is corporeal continuity, so there is a *psychological continuity*. I have already mentioned the delay in the apprehension of the dead person, which finds expression in the attitudes towards the dead person. It is natural to show respect or even awe for the dead.

There is also what could be called a *symbolic continuity* between the living person and the dead one. Sometimes a portrait (often a photograph), perhaps with a candle or a flower, is shown at the funeral service. The relation between the living person and her portrait is a symbolic one. The portrait represents the person in an important sense. The same goes for the graveyard and the tombstone. The continuity is so strong that an act of disrespect with regard to the portrait or the grave is experienced as disrespect for the person herself.

The dead person is present in a remarkable sense during the funeral service and during the social gathering that usually follows. This is a kind of psychological and symbolic presence. She is so to speak more 'alive' or present during these times than ever. This has to do with the synchronic context of the life story of the dead person. Relatives and friends remember her.

So there is both a corporeal and a mental continuity between the person as alive and as dead. The mental continuity is certainly not *intrapersonal*. As far as we know there cannot be a link of memories between the living and the dead person. But there is an *interpersonal* continuity. The dead person is part of a coherent chain of memories in other people. She is part of a common life story.

I know of several cases where someone who has lost their partner, especially an older person, often speaks to their deceased husband or wife. There is a certain reticence about this; people tend to be embarrassed about it, although it seems to be a rather common and natural phenomenon. When we have been used to sharing impressions and experiences with another person for a long time in daily life, it is quite natural to see and hear and witness what happens together with that person even after her death. We experience the world around as it were with the eyes and ears of our partner, and this might give rise to a kind of tacit or even audible dialogue.

8.4   The necessary psychological change

There is normally a change in the view of the dead person, from the apprehension of her in her bodily reality to remembering her. An experienced hospice doctor told me that only once in her long professional career had she been asked by a dying patient, 'What will happen to my body after death?' This patient obviously wanted to know details about the handling of her body after her death. I suspect that there is a natural tendency to push aside speculations about the decay of the body after death. For the dying person, and still more for their relatives, it is essential to change the point of view. From the moment of death we want to change our focus from the decaying body to the memory of the person. Perhaps the need for this change of perspective is not only natural but even necessary for the mourning process. And the funeral, not least the social gathering, is a time of change. Face to face with the grave we normally tend to contemplate the memory of the deceased and not her gradual bodily decay.

8.5   Brain death as a special category

Today the borderline between life and death has been altered by the introduction of the modern brain-related concept of death, and we may encounter a situation where the patient is dead according to the new concept but presents some characteristics of a living person such as a complexion with normal skin colour, a beating heart and a chest that rises for breath (although with artificial help from the ventilator). Such a state of brain death, made possible by advanced medical technology, may last some time. This state provides new possibilities of organ donation and transplantation. Let us call this exceptional state *brain death* (meaning death together with artificial respiration and heartbeat) in contrast to *ordinary death* (a state that of course includes the death of the brain).

In what sense is brain death a special category of death? It is a fact that we seem to see a living person, even though we intellectually understand that the person is dead. Therefore a reductionist view of the brain-dead person is more difficult to apply than in respect of the ordinary dead person.

Legally there is no difference between the brain dead and the ordinary dead in so far as the same legal rules apply when it comes to official declaration of death, inheritance, etc. But in the preparatory work for the Swedish legislation regarding the concept of death there are some specific provisions for the handling of the brain dead (SOU 1984:79). There it states that medical treatment ought to cease at the moment of death, i.e. when all activities of the brain have ceased. This is justified by the principle of medical utility and also by considerations of economy. Medical utility (and medical futility) has to do with medical experience and clinical skill. I understand this as a reference to traditional medical clinical ethics. But three exceptions are allowed for (SOU 1984:79, pp. 301–303):

- When treatment, including artificial heart stimulation and ventilation necessary for the harvesting of organs for transplantation, is called for.
- When a brain-dead woman is at a late stage of pregnancy.
- When relatives should be given some time to accept the death. In this case, it is acknowledged that for religious, psychological or ethical reasons relatives may find it difficult to accept brain death.

The preparatory work admits that the concept of brain death opens the possibility of 'post-mortem examination under ventilation in progress' but is hesitant about it (for ethical reasons, obviously). The suggestion is that this case and the aforementioned three exceptions do not demand special legislation. They are left to clinical ethical decision-making.

Thus for me it is obvious that brain death is seen as a special category of death. There are specific ethical problems connected with it. Or, if you like, there are specific ethical considerations to be taken into account. Even if a brain-dead person might be the optimal specimen for educational or research purposes, such a use seems to be morally objectionable.

8.6   Fear of the dead person

Fear of the dead person should be distinguished from the fear of death (which in turn can be understood either as a fear of dying or a fear of being dead), although those fears may influence a person's fear of the dead person. There are indications that a fear of dead people is common, and my interviews confirm this.

In Sweden today many patients want to stay at home when they are seriously ill, and this is made possible by different forms of home care. Even advanced medical treatment is available in a patient's own home, and advanced care can be delivered until the end of life. But sometimes a patient who has been cared for at home still wants to be taken to hospital at the very end of life.

I was told about an elderly couple sitting watching TV. Suddenly the man said: 'I feel ill. I think I'm going to die'. Very quickly he was taken to hospital and within 48 hours he died there. The wife's comment was interesting: 'What luck that we got to the hospital in time!' How can this reaction be explained? Would it not have been better for the man to die in peace and quiet at home with his wife? One reason might be that she wanted her husband to have the opportunity of treatment that might perhaps have saved his life. Another reason might be that by having him cared for in hospital she was spared from the responsibility. But there might also have been a feeling of appropriateness; death belongs to the hospital context; that's the place for dying. Or was she simply afraid of having him at home, dead?

The ideal might be to stay at home at the end of life. But when somebody is actually lying dead at home there is a change of perspective. You are accustomed to caring for a family member, often during a long period of illness, and now you are confronted with the new situation of having a dead person nearby. Social services home care staff report a great fear of coming to a home and finding a person dead. One might think that the prospect of finding somebody severely ill would be worse than finding a person lying dead, but obviously this is not always the case. I have been told of very brave and capable people who have been grateful that their partner reached the hospital in time and did not die at home, otherwise they could not think of staying in the flat or house, or at least not in the room where the person died. One of my informants, a clergyman, told me of a Roma family who had declined to rent a flat because a person had recently died there.

Are there any rational motives for such a fear? Medically there are not. The dead body does not present any threat to other people. The body is unlikely to be contagious. Still, there are strong taboos concerning the dead body.

The Swedish psychologist Margareta Sanner has investigated people's reasons for feeling discomfort about being examined post-mortem (Sanner 1992, p. 69). Her results are shown in Table 8.1.

The most frequent answer refers to discomfort about being cut up after death. If this is understood as a fear of feeling discomfort although dead, it is irrational or even absurd. But a more probable interpretation is that it is about a discomfort we feel, while alive, about being dissected when dead. If so, it is no stranger than the idea that we have a reasonable interest in what happens to us after death. This is in line with the idea that the living have interests and rights which reach beyond the moment of death. This reason for discomfort seems to overlap with the answer referring to lack of respect for the dead. Taken together, these reasons are mentioned by over 62% of the interviewees.

Fear of not being really dead is the second most common answer, given by an average 34% of those asked about their reasons for discomfort about being examined

Table 8.1 Reasons for feeling uncomfortable about the idea of a post-mortem examination

Reason	Age		
	18–25 years (n = 465)	30–59 years (n = 345)	60–75 years (n = 97)
Discomfort about being cut up after death	51%	38%	33%
Afraid of not being really dead	29%	41%	32%
Lack of respect for the dead	25%	17%	24%
Worry about medical progress	12%	12%	14%
Think that relatives are against it	13%	8%	12%
Mistrust of health care	10%	9%	5%
Do not want to reveal one's illness	4%	6%	11%
It is against nature	5%	3%	8%
Can affect resurrection	8%	5%	3%
Can affect funeral	8%	3%	6%
It is against God's will	3%	3%	9%
Other feelings of discomfort	7%	5%	2%

post-mortem. Historically, the fear of mistakes about apparent death has played an important role. It probably has its roots in a society before modern medicine with its diagnostic facilities, but paradoxically it has had something of a comeback in recent times when the concept of death has been revisited because of the need for transplants (see earlier). A brain-related concept of death presupposes very advanced diagnostic techniques, so there might be fear of mistakes when it comes to so-called brain death.

It is interesting to note that very few respondents refer to purely religious motives. The answers that emphasise religious reasons, referring to resurrection and God's will, amount to only a little more than 10% in total.

8.7 The rights of the dead

Can the dead have rights? In order to answer this question we first need to decide what we mean by a right. In this context I do not merely mean right in the sense that an act or an attitude is right or morally appropriate. I will use the concept of a right in the strong sense of a claim-right (Hohfeld 1964). A right in this sense is connected with a duty either normatively or conceptually. A right is *normatively* connected with a duty if there is a moral or legal obligation to fulfil the right. A right is *conceptually* or logically connected with a duty if part of the meaning of the right is connected with the duty. In both cases we may talk of a strong right. We can further distinguish between legal and moral rights in this strong sense.

I take it that the so-called human rights, for instance as specified in the UN Charter, are moral rights whereas the rights that normally appear in a legal system are legal rights. A moral right can be justified by moral reasons. A moral justification of a right can be in terms of a general moral consensus or in terms of some kind of normative moral theory such as in forms of utilitarianism or in Kantianism or some other moral theory.

Rights may be *in rem* rights or *in personam* rights. The former is a right that holds in relation to everybody and the latter is a right in relation to a specific person. Rights of animals or of newborn babies or of people with severe intellectual disabilities may be asymmetrical, so that the animal, the baby or the person has rights but no duties. Nevertheless the right of the animal, the baby or the person is connected with duties, albeit duties of other moral beings, and is thus a right of the *in rem* kind.

So far I have taken rights in a generic sense, i.e. as rights in general. But we need to distinguish between moral and legal rights. Moral and legal rights as well as norms differ both in form and in justification. The main formal difference has to do with the institutionalisation of legal rights and norms. That is to say, the legal right is publicly promulgated, it is handled by certain authorities and normally connected with sanctions settled beforehand (in legislation or in case law). These are important conditions for what is called the *rule of law* (German *Rechtssicherheit*, Swedish *rättssäkerhet*). It is foreseeable how a right to something will be realised. Rule of law is a kind of meta-law, and represents an important social value. Moral rights, on the other hand, are not institutionalised in this manner. They are informal.

Moral and legal rights also differ when it comes to their justification. On one level a legal right is justified by the very fact that it is valid within a certain legal system. The validity of a right may be explained either as following from a hierarchy of legal statutes, or as being normally vindicated by legal authorities in a legal system. The so-called theory of pure jurisprudence (German *reine Rechtslehre*) set forth by the Austrian legal philosopher Hans Kelsen is a theory of the former kind and Scandinavian positivism is a theory of the latter kind. But on a moral and more fundamental level a legal right is justified by being the outcome of a democratic decision-making procedure.

What is the relation between (justified) legal and moral norms or rights? Generally speaking, moral norms play an important role in respect of legal norms. Typically the enactment of a law comes about after moral considerations. Moral considerations also play a role when it comes to the administration of the enactment. The relations between legal and moral rights can be characterised as congruent, conflicting or complimentary.

- Normally there is a *congruency* between a legal norm or right and its corresponding moral norm or right. For instance, in most legal systems there are norms forbidding assault corresponding to moral norms forbidding maltreatment. But for several reasons there need not be a complete congruency between all legal norms and their corresponding moral norms. First, not every immoral act can be forbidden in law. That would lead to an intolerably legalistic society. Second, moral norms can and should often be more rigorous, more demanding, than their equivalent legal norms. Complete congruency is neither possible nor desirable.
- Legal and moral norms or rights may *conflict*. A conflict of this kind gives rise to a problem. Sometimes, but not always, the moral norm in such cases should have priority. The case for civil disobedience for moral reasons presents a serious conflict. An open society leaves some room for avoiding the conflict by refraining from taking legal measures or by setting up provisions for exceptional individual cases.

- Since, as just said, moral norms may be more demanding than their legal counter-parts, the relation between the two kinds of norms or rights may be one of *complementarity*. That is, the moral norm exceeds the legal norm.

In what sense, then, can the dead have rights? First, the living person may have rights that reach beyond the moment of her death. This is so both for legal and for moral rights. That is why the legal system normally respects testamentary provisions; there are legal rules for the execution of a will. There is also a moral consensus of respect for a person's wishes when it comes to the handling of her body after death. For instance, it is desirable for many reasons for a person to leave instructions about her future funeral. It may be a relief for the relatives to know about such wishes, since we normally want to comply with them and thus honour the dead person.

Such rights for the living person are, so to speak, transmitted to the dead, and there is nothing controversial or mysterious about this. But in my view the dead as such also may have rights. This may seem more controversial. Does not having a right presuppose having wishes? And a wish is obviously a psychic act that the dead cannot be said to exercise. Now, this objection can be understood in two ways.

First, there is the view that the right-holder must be able to express her right or at least imagine her right. But this is unreasonable. I may have a right to something, e.g. to an inheritance, even if I am not aware of it, or if I am asleep or unconscious. A person with severe intellectual disability or mental illness has rights. The same goes for other living creatures such as animals. The idea that having a right presupposes having a specific wish is an example of a kind of psycho-logistic thought confusing certain psychic acts with the content of the concept of a right.

Second, there is the view that one must be able to vindicate one's right in order to possess it. But this is not true. A right may be ineffective because no one vindicates it, for instance brings it to court. But the right is still there. I may have a right to something, for instance to a certain kind of medical treatment, without trying to enforce it (or even without bothering about it or being aware of it).

Another objection to the view that the dead as such have rights is that rights presuppose needs and that a dead person cannot have needs. In my view there can be rights that do not presuppose needs. For instance, you may have a right to some economic compensation without being in need of it. But it is also true that a need is often an important moral justification of a right.

What, then, is a need? A need is what is required according to some standard normal functioning. Consider the following examples:

Man needs love.

The horse needs feeding.

The tree needs water.

The roof needs repairing.

In the generic sense a need is what is necessary or indispensable for attaining a specific goal. The goal might be biological, aesthetic, pragmatic and so forth. That is to say, a need does not have to be a human need or even a natural need. In this sense 'need'

'stands simply for any necessary condition for the attaining of a goal' A need is dependent on contextual factors such as social conventions, traditions, etc. (Nordenfelt 1995,
pp. 58–65).

The three first of the above-mentioned assertions refer to biological or natural needs.
The last one, on the other hand, refers to a conventional or aesthetic need according to
some understanding of normal or aesthetic function. The needs of the dead seem to
belong to this category. So, for instance, the need of the dead person for respect and
reverence is a need grounded in a cultural convention about how to treat her. The dead
person has needs, and needs are important for the moral justification of a right. This
brings us back to the question of the moral justification of the rights of the dead.

So far I have demonstrated that there are no conceptual obstacles to the existence of
rights of the dead. I have also discussed the general justification of legal rights (or
norms). On one level there are justifications of the validity of legal rights, either from
higher legal norms in the hierarchy of a legal system or from the very effectiveness of
the rights. On a more basic level, in a democratic society the legal system itself is justified by its being the outcome of a democratic decision-making process and the outcome
of what is commonly called the ideal of the rule of law.

Now there are also justifications for specific legal rights. They often appear during
the preparatory work for legislation, where moral and public interests are given as a
reason for the proposed legal provision. That is so because the normal relation between
legal and moral rights or norms is one of congruence or complementarity. So there is
a need for a moral justification of the specific legislation.

This brings us back to the question of the justification of moral rights. How can the
rights, legal or moral, of the dead be morally justified? I assume that they can be justified either from a general normative theory or from a pragmatic combination of different kinds of moral principles.

Different forms of utilitarianism present different problems when it comes to the
justification of rights of the dead. According to *act utilitarianism* the calculation of utility
should be made for every single problematic choice of action. Irrespective of whether
utility is understood as a maximum of pleasure or welfare or as a maximum of preference realisation, the calculation of utility in every single case may result in different
evaluations of a right. That is to say, the outcome will vary depending on specific circumstances. So, act utilitarianism, whether preferential or hedonistic, will hardly result
in the justification of strong individual rights.

Rule utilitarianism, on the other hand, can justify such strong individual rights, since
there might be good reason for assuming that a right will be conducive to a positive
balance of welfare or preference realisation. For instance, adherence to the wishes of a
person regarding her treatment after death could be justified from considerations of the
well-being (or preferences) of all living persons involved.

The rights of the dead may also be morally justified from a *contractarian* moral theory.
Then it could be assumed that people in a given society would accept such rights since
they are taken to be in the interest of all informed and rational members of the society.

I take it that the legislator and the public in a given society will seldom accede to a
single specific normative theory when it comes to their justification of a single specific
right of the dead. In real life they will rather adhere to a mix of principles, values and
considerations of different kinds. Probably they will put forward values such as piety,

integrity and benevolence, and refer to tradition, habit and religious convictions. Such a more or less pragmatic mix of considerations could justify for them specific rights of the dead. Actually, among my interviewees I have found no example of an attempt to justify the rights of the dead from any single explicit normative theory.

8.8   Who owns the dead?

The dead person is a legal object (German *Rechtsobjekt*) but not a legal subject (German *Rechtssubjekt*). That is to say, the estate of the deceased person is a legal subject, which can raise claims in court (i.e. partners in the estate of the deceased may raise claims on behalf of the estate), but the estate is distinct from the dead person. The estate of the deceased person is hardly the owner of the body of the dead person. So it seems relevant to ask who is the owner of the body of the dead person.

One standard answer is that the dead person is the property of the hospital and ultimately of the principal of the hospital, in Sweden typically the county council. But this answer rests on a simplification. It is necessary to take a closer look at the concept of property (Lantz 1977, pp. 24–31). A property right has two dimensions: (1) tenure (secured possession) and (2) freedom of disposition. The ideal type (in Max Weber's sense) of property comprises full tenure and total freedom of disposition. But this ideal type is never realised in any legal system. Instances of property right in a legal system, the real types (again in Max Weber's sense), always consist of limited tenure and freedom of disposal. They can be placed on a scale from zero to full realisation of these dimensions.

The tenure, the secured possession of the dead person, is divided between the relatives and the hospital, religious authorities and other actors. Nobody can disturb the possession without the consent of any of these actors. The tenure in itself is very strong. The freedom of disposition, on the other hand, is very limited. It is restricted by many legal (as well as moral) norms. What might be done to the body of the dead person is clearly specified by traditional, moral as well as legal restrictions. As a matter of fact, very few measures can be taken with regard to the dead. Hospitals have very strict routines. Relatives have a certain freedom of choice between forms of funeral. The freedom of possession can, like the tenure, be seen as divided between the different actors. So if we want to speak of a property right regarding the dead, it is in fact a very restricted property right.

8.9   Religious aspects

'From time immemorial taking care that the bodies of the dead do not lie unburied has been seen as a holy duty among all nationalities. The sense of piety has required this' (Schmidt 1920, pp. 249–251). Although the ways of caring for the deceased person have varied widely across periods and cultures it has always and everywhere been a duty to perform such care, and not being decently buried or burned (or whatever has been the cultural custom) has been looked upon as the source of great shame. This duty has been of a moral kind and always connected with religious ideas. In fact, most practices concerning the handling of the dead have been performed in a religious ritual setting. Even in very secularised countries, as in northern Europe today, purely non-religious funerals are in the minority. That is probably so because the view of the dead presupposes notions of the human race and its destiny. What I have called a thananthropology is grounded in anthropology. The fact of death gives rise to questions of life and its limits and of future life (eschatology). In all religions the funeral practices are linked to the future fate of the dead. They aim to prepare the dead person for her future life.

The main forms of funeral throughout history have been burial in the ground and burning. In the three monotheistic religions, Judaism, Christendom and Islam, burial has dominated. Not until in the 20th century was burning (cremation) introduced in Christian societies. The Catholic church has not accepted this practice, and it first met with resistance in Protestant churches too. In the 21st century it has become a practice of the same importance as burial in some Protestant churches (for instance, in Sweden and the UK). Burning of the dead has been the general practice in Hindu India.

Other forms of funeral exist. For instance, the setting out of the dead body is the tradition in Zoroastriansm with its roots in ancient Persia. The dead person is set out in a 'tower of silence' where vultures or other animals eat her. In Zoroastrian thought it is important that the corpse should not pollute the elements.

Mummification may also be mentioned. We know it from ancient Egypt, but it can be practised in other religions too. For instance, in Palermo in Sicily there is a catacomb connected to a Capuchin monastery where mummified bodies are exposed still wearing their customary clothing. This practice existed in Palermo from 1599 until 1880. The eating of body parts of the dead, i.e. cannibalism, has been practised in the South Pacific as part of the funeral.

In every culture and every religion the treatment of the dead is characterised by a dual attitude: reverence and awe on one hand and fear on the other. A typical example of the fear of the dead in Judaeo-Christian thought is to be found in the New Testament (Matthew 23, 27, King James version): 'Woe unto you, scribes and Pharisees, hypocrites! Ye are like unto whited sepulchres, which indeed appear beautiful outward, but are within full of dead men's bones, and of all uncleanness'. This reflects the Judean fear of the impurity of the dead. Tombs used to be lime-washed as a sign and a warning. In later Christian thought there has been not only this idea of a kind of taboo, difficult to explain rationally, but also a fear of spectres, i.e. a fear of the dead person coming back as a ghost because she has not found rest and peace in the grave.

The attitude of reverence and awe is evident in all cultures and religions irrespective of whether the funeral takes the form of burial or setting out, or even includes cannibalism. They are all signs of respect and veneration. The idea is, according to (among others) Emile Durkheim, to strengthen the bond between the living and the dead. The funeral is therefore often associated with a ritual meal. In the Christian tradition Holy Communion exemplifies this. The attitudes of fear and awe are universal.

Let me briefly focus on the Judaeo-Christian view of death and the dead. In the Old Testament Man is seen as a whole, with no sharp distinction between the mental and physical aspects. Soul (*nefesch*) is a vital aspect of the body but not a separate entity. The anthropology of the Old Testament is holistic. Death is the natural end of human life. It is not seen as a punishment, although too early a death might be seen as a misfortune or even a punishment for sin. Death is followed by a shadowy existence in the

Kingdom of Death. 'For in death there is no remembrance of thee; in the grave who shall give thee thanks?' (Psalms 6, 5). The dead body is looked upon as impure, but this does not exclude reverence and piety in relation to the dead person. The hope of a continued personal existence after death, an individual future life, appears late in the Old Testament scriptures.

In the New Testament the fact of death and the hope of an eternal life are central. The death of Jesus is described as preceded by his agony in Gethsemane and on the cross. It is a harsh and painful death, but it is followed by his resurrection on the third day. In Pauline theology the life and deeds of Christ are depicted as a vicarious victory over death.

According to New Testament eschatology Man is predestined after death to meet God on the Day of Judgement. Resurrection means judgement. The verdict will be either eternal punishment or blessedness in communion with God. The idea of punishment especially has inspired iconography and popular fantasy from the Middle Ages until our own time. St Thomas Aquinas distinguished between punishment as separation from God (*poena damni*) and punishment as corporeal punishment (*poena sensus*) (Aquinas 1948). In the *Divina Commedia* Dante combined these two ideas by depicting the punishment in Hell as a state where the sinner remains, as it were, frozen in his evil will, and the punishment therefore consists in the eternal continuation of the sin that separates him from God. So, for Dante, punishment is self-inflicted. In mediaeval thought, for example in the *Paradiso* of the *Divina Commedia*, eternal blessedness is less vividly depicted, since it consists in the more abstract idea of a full realisation of human potentialities in communion with God. The underlying idea of both states is that after death no more human decisions are possible.

How does life continue after death according to Christian theology? In 1959 the French theologian Oscar Cullman revived an old theologian debate concerning this question (Cullmann 1959). For Cullmann there is a clear difference between a philosophical belief in immortality and a Christian belief in resurrection. The former is said to reflect ancient Greek ideas of an immortal soul grounded in a dualistic view, where body and material are seen as unclean and evil, whereas the soul represents the clean and spiritual element (Rohde 1925). Only the soul has a share of the divine substance. In Cullmann's view only the belief in the resurrection of the flesh is in accordance with the biblical, holistic, view of Man. This understanding of resurrection (*resurrectio carnis*) is set out in the Apostolic Creed (*credo in … resurrectionem carnis*). In popular Christianity both ideas – eternal life of the soul and resurrection of the dead – exist side by side. This goes for both Roman Catholic and Protestant theology.

There is a great distance between academic theology and popular practice, and one should not expect to find very articulate ideas behind popular practices. According to my informants, especially among the younger generation, there is now great symbolic creativity when it comes to funerals. It is very common to put personal belongings and souvenirs in the coffin with the dead body. Even a bottle of the dead person's favourite wine or whisky may be placed there – or favourite toys, in the case of a child. The dead person may be dressed in her working clothes or her wedding dress. This is certainly not to be understood as a sign of a belief in corporeal resurrection, but rather as a symbolic act.

Nor are traditional common practices such as opening the windows after the moment of death to be taken as a proof of a well-thought-out belief in an eternal surviving soul.

183

The same goes for conversing with the loved one after her or his death. This seems to be very common, although people are reluctant to speak of it, probably because it is thought of as irrational or even as a sign of mental illness, although as mentioned above it is psychologically very understandable. But you cannot invoke this phenomenon to draw conclusions about elaborate ideas of a surviving soul.

I have referred to a general human tradition of caring for and showing respect for the dead. There seems to be a duty to show respect for the dead. I have also said that this care is almost always linked to religious beliefs and practised in religious ritual settings. Now, are there specific religious justifications for the right of the dead to be met with respect and piety? I have said that one reason for this right and corresponding duty is the religious imperative to prepare for the future of the dead. If we turn to the Western Christian context, we can ask whether there are any typically Christian justifications for the rights of the dead.

First, there is the argument from Judaeo-Christian anthropology. From a Judaeo-Christian perspective, Man is the creation of God. When creation is described in Genesis 1, 10–25, day by day, every verse ends with the statement 'and God saw that it was good'. The entire creation is holy, sacred, since it is created and intended by God.

Second, there is the argument from *imago Dei*. 'God said, let us make man in our image, after our likeness; and let them have dominion over the fish of the sea, and over the fowl of the air, and over the cattle, and over all the earth, and over every creeping thing that creepeth upon the earth' (Genesis 1, 26). God-likeliness is usually interpreted as implying a stewardship and a moral responsibility for the rest of the creation. This gives Man a very important position and role.

Third, there is the argument from soteriology, i.e. from God's plan for salvation. Man has a role in God's eternal plan. Man is the object of God's love, and Man is intended by God to attain communion with him.

Fourth, there is a theological argument. St Paul writes, 'your body is the temple of the Holy Ghost' (1 Corinthians 6, 19). If in Hebrew thought the body and everything material is clean and good (because it is God's creation) and if in Hellenistic thought the material is seen as evil and opposed to the higher soul, then in Pauline theology the body as such is neither good nor evil, neither pure nor impure, but the body of the Christian is, so to speak, possessed by Christ and consequently a holy temple.

The first two kinds of justification for the special rights of the body are common Judaeo-Christian trains of thought, whereas the other two are specifically Christian (although the third one concerns everybody and the fourth concerns only Christians).

So much for the religious, especially the Judaeo-Christian, aspect of the dead. Let us briefly turn to the agnostic and atheist aspect. In Western Europe many people do not believe in a monotheistic faith (Christian, Jewish or Muslim). We can assume that there are among these people those who have a well-thought-out agnostic or atheist conviction. There are also quite a number of people who have a more or less vague belief in some Supreme Power. At least for atheists there cannot be a personal life after death. However, a belief in reincarnation is not a rare thing today – a belief that is foreign to Christian, Jewish and Muslim theology.

I want to distinguish between two levels of ideas about the dead. First, elaborate theological ideas acknowledged in a religion or church. Second, popular ideas among adherents of a religion or church. There might be a big gap between those two. For instance, the theological debate, referred to above, concerning whether the survival of the soul or the resurrection of the body should be seen as the genuine Christian doctrine is probably unknown to most members of Christian churches, but my supposition is that among ordinary church members the belief in a surviving soul is predominant.

On the level of practice we can find a multitude of habits and customs in relation to the dead. I have already referred to the wide ranges of forms the funeral may take. Even though burial and cremation are the predominant forms of funeral in Christian society today, there are many variants. After cremation the ashes might be buried in an urn in an individual grave, or the urn can be placed in a columbarium, or the ashes can be scattered in a memorial park, or over a particular area of land or at sea.

The funeral most often follows a religious ritual, but the range of individual variations is wide. Ministers and undertakers have told me that the symbolic creativity is great, especially among younger people. A special case is the increase during the AIDS epidemic at the beginning of the 1990s of imaginative and very personal funerals among the gay community. However, it is risky to use these various and highly individual funeral practices to make inferences about any underlying religious convictions or ideas about the future fate of the dead.

Holm & Lahtinen (1985) interviewed people about their choice between burial and cremation. Most interviewees referred to tradition or emotional reasons; only 4% referred to religious convictions (Holm & Lahtinen 1985, p. 27). Although tradition and emotion may stand for many different kinds of thoughts, it is obvious that few people justified their choice by elaborate theological reasons.

Dahlgren and Hermansson (see Dahlgren & Gustafsson 2006, p. 54) have created a typology for funerals, distinguishing lay and church components on an institutional and an individual level respectively (Table 8.2).

Dahlgren and Hermansson have not gone further with a quantitative study. It is clear, though, that in Sweden a great majority of funeral services take place in a church (types a and b). From my own experience and from reports from my informants I assume that a considerable number of funerals should be categorised as type b.

Purely secular funerals (type d) are uncommon in Sweden, although they are reported to be increasing in number. In one extreme form of secular funeral, almost a kind of

Table 8.2 Typology for funerals

		Individual level Do individuals show any belief in an existence beyond the present?	
		Yes	No
Institutional level Is the funeral performed according to an established rule or ritual?	Yes	a. Funeral service	b. Funeral service
	No	c. Secular funeral with religious components	d. Secular funeral

185

non-funeral, the ashes of the dead person are taken directly to a cemetery after cremation without any ceremony, either religious or secular. The number of such funerals is
uncertain, but one estimate (Dahlgren & Gustafsson 2006, p. 20) is that there are approximately 1000 of them per year in Sweden (about 1% of all funerals).

8.10   The dignity of the dead

Human dignity is the basis for human rights. The preamble of the UN Declaration of
Human Rights recognises 'the inherent dignity … of all members of the human family'.
Thus, dignity is a moral concept implying certain basic rights. We have analysed the
concept of dignity as referring to four aspects: (1) dignity of merit, (2) dignity as moral
stature, (3) the dignity of identity and (4) human dignity or *Menschenwürde* (Nordenfelt
2003, 2004). It is obvious that the UN Charter concerns living human beings. How far
can the concept of dignity in its different components be said to apply to the dead? In
what sense (or senses) can the dead be said to have dignity?

8.10.1   Dignity of merit
First, there is a formal dignity of merit. For instance, a member of the royal family or
an archbishop has a dignity in this sense. After death a member of the royal family
often lies in state. That is, she, or rather her coffin, is exposed in a solemn and ceremoni-
ous way, with a military guard. This is an occasion intended for the public veneration
of the royal person. The tomb of a member of royalty or of a bishop or of some other
dignitary used to be a place to show reverence, a place for piety. A clerical dignitary
may be buried within the walls of a church.

Second, there is an informal dignity of merit. Saints, for example, are the objects of
veneration after death. Their tombs are sites for adoration or even worship. Especially
in Catholic tradition parts of the body of saints, so-called relics, may be kept in the altar
of a church.

It is common for a gravestone to be inscribed not only with the name of the deceased
but also with her title or (in older times) with the abbreviations of honours conferred
upon her. So it is obvious that people after death may be looked upon with a dignity
of merit, formal or informal.

8.10.2   Dignity as moral stature
The dignity of merit of a deceased person, as described above, may have a moral basis.
This is especially the case for saints, and for many non-religious heroes as well.

The treatment of the dead person according to their moral stature can be exemplified
by the tradition in olden times of burying criminals or people who had committed
suicide outside the churchyard or on the north side of the church. An extreme case is
the humiliation of the body of Benito Mussolini, the former dictator of Italy, which was
dragged around hanging upside down on a truck.

As mentioned earlier, the evaluation of a person may change over time. The former
Indian sovereign Zafar, who was also a Sufi mystic and poet, was dethroned and ban-
ished for his association with the Sepoy uprising against the British in India in 1857. As
late as 1991 his grave was found and is now venerated as a holy place.

8.10.3   The dignity of identity

The two former kinds of dignity may vary considerably between people. The merit or moral stature of a dead person may even have a negative value, which may be reflected in non-dignity of merit or moral stature. These kinds of dignity are the object of changing attitudes and evaluation. Even the dignity of identity can be hurt and diminished, but it still pertains to every human being. Everyone is entitled to dignity of identity because every human being is the subject of their unique life world, and consequently the centre and main figure of a life world.

I have already said that the identity of a person is not only her corporeal identity but also what we could call her narrative identity. That is to say, a person has her identity as a life story, and this narrative identity has a diachronic as well as a synchronic aspect. So the identity must be related to the social context of the person as well as to her personal history.

How, then, can the dignity of identity of the dead in this sense be hurt or diminished? First, the corporeal dignity of the dead may of course be damaged. Offences against the body of the dead person can easily be exemplified. In every legal system there are prohibitions against interfering in an unauthorised and insulting way with the dead. Such crimes as necrophilia and desecration of a grave are well known. Second, the narrative identity of the dead may be infringed. Calumny against a living person is a crime that has, at least morally, an equivalent regarding the dead. The dead can be violated by verbal offences such as slander and lies. We sometimes say that the memory of the person is violated. As for dignity of merit and moral stature, even the dignity of identity of a person, may change over time. If the dignity of identity of the living person is to some extent a symmetrical relation between that person and other people, the relation between the dead person and other people is an asymmetric one, where the dead person cannot defend herself against accusations, misinterpretations and slander, so the moral obligation to respect the dignity of the dead person is even stronger. There is the Latin saying *de mortuis nil nisi bonum* (say nothing but good about the dead). If the narrative identity of the dead person is misinterpreted in a malicious way, it may also hurt her family and relatives.

Dignity of identity is not only about feelings, as noted by Nordenfelt (2004), but about something more objective, at least about something intersubjective. A person, alive or dead, can be hurt without her knowing it. To speak ill of a person behind her back without her knowing it is to hurt her and is consequently an immoral act.

On the other hand, the dignity of a dead person can be restored. It happens whenever her memory is kept in awe and her life and deeds are spoken of and interpreted in a kind and benevolent way. To forget a dead relative may be an insult. But to remember her and cultivate her memory and her grave is tantamount to maintaining her dignity of identity. In many cultures this is an important duty, but whether it is an actual duty in today's Western world can be questioned.

8.10.4   Human dignity (*Menschenwürde*)

This kind of dignity is due to every living human being and cannot be diminished. The idea of a general human dignity is deep-rooted in Western thought. Historically it has religious roots and goes back to Judaeo-Christian theology (see Religious aspects, above). Still there are older, non-Christian ideas in the same vein. In Stoic philosophy

187

there is the idea of the *scintilla animae*, the spark of divineness, inherent in every human being.

As noted by Nordenfelt (2004), the idea of a general human dignity is difficult to justify on secular grounds although the idea is fundamental to a modern welfare society. Further, the idea of a general human dignity as well as the idea of human rights is primarily applicable to living persons. What does it means in terms of dignity and rights for the dead?

First, there is a derived or secondary dignity of the dead. That is, the dead person has been a human being with full human dignity. This fact is mirrored in the dignity and the right to piety that pertains to her.

Second, there is an equality face to face with death. This goes for both the dying person and for the dead person. An attitude of respect, sympathy and compassion is due to the dying person. Death is common to all living beings. Face to face with death we experience our own mortality and our own anxiety. We share the same fate. And to this extent we are all equal in dignity.

References

Aquinas, St Thomas (1948) *Summa Theologiae Ia–IIae, q. 87:4 resp.* Christian Classics, Complete English edition. Vol. 2, pp. 975–976. Ave Maria Press, Notre Dame, IL.

Brecher, B. (2002) Our obligation to the dead. *Journal of Applied Philosophy*, **19**, 109–119.

Cullmann, O. (1959) *Immortalité de l'âme ou résurrection des morts? [Immortality of the soul or resurrection of the dead?]* Delachaux and Niestlé, Neuchatel.

Dahlgren, C. & Gustafsson, G. (eds) (2006) *Kring begravningar i nutid: tre studier [On funerals in present times: three studies].* Lund Studies in Sociology of Religion, **6**, Lund.

Dahlgren, C. & Hermansson, J. (2006) 'Här skall min aska vila'; nya platser och riter för gravsättning av aska på andra platser än begravningsplats. ['Here my ashes shall rest'; new places and rites for burying ashes in other places than at a cemetery]. In: *Kring begravningar i nutid: tre studier* (eds C. Dahlgren & G. Gustafsson), pp. 7–56. Lund Studies in Sociology of Religion, **6**, Lund.

Hohfeld, W.N. (1964) *Fundamental Legal Conceptions as Applied in Judicial Reasoning.* Yale University Press, New Haven, CT (orginally published in 1919).

Holm, N.G. & Lahtinen, T. (1985) *Jordbegravning eller kremering? En studie av gravskicket i Finland. [Burial or cremation? A study of funeral customs in Finland].* Åbo Akademi, Turku.

Lantz, G. (1977) *Eigentumsrecht – ein Recht oder ein Unrecht* [Property right – a right or a wrong]. Acta Universitatis Upsaliensis; Uppsala Studies in Social Ethics, No 4; Almqvist & Wiksell International, Stockholm.

Lantz, G. (1997) *Vårdetik; berättelsen om Arthur* [Health-care ethics; the story of Arthur]. Liber AB, Stockholm (first published in 1992).

Moritz, M. (1970) Über den Begriff der juristischen Person [On the concept of the legal person]. In: *Proceedings of the XIVth International Congress of Philosophy*, pp. 113–131. University of Vienna, Vienna.

Nordenfelt, L. (1995) *On the Nature of Health*, 2nd, revised, edition, Kluwer, Dordrecht.

Nordenfelt, L. (2000) *Action, Ability, and Health.* Kluwer, Dordrecht.

Nordenfelt, L. (2003) Dignity of the elderly: an introduction. *Medicine, Health Care, and Philosophy*, **6**, 99–101.

Nordenfelt, L. (2004) Varieties of dignity. *Health Care Analysis*, **12**, 69–81.

Nozick, R. (1990) *Examined Life: Philosophical Meditations*. Simon and Schuster, New York.

Rohde, E. (1925) *Psyche; Seelencult und Unsterblichkeitsglaube der Griechen* [The cult of souls and belief in immortality among the Greeks], 9th edn (1st edn 1894). J.C.B. Mohr, Tübingen.

Sanner, M. (1992) *Den sista undersökningen – obduktion i ett psykologiskt perspektiv* [The last examination – autopsy from a psychological perspective]. SOU 1992:17. Allmänna Förlaget, Stockholm.

Schmidt, V. (1920) Begravelsen [funeral]. In: *Kirkeleksikon for Norden* [Church dictionary for Scandinavia] (ed. F. Nielsen), pp. 249–251. Jydsk Forlagsforretning, Copenhagen.

SOU (1984:79) *Dödsbegreppet; huvudbetänkande från Utredningen om dödsbegreppet* [Swedish Government Official Report: *The concept of death*]. Ministry of Social Affairs, Stockholm.

Taylor, C. (1985) *Philosophical Papers, Vol. 2: Philosophy and the Human Sciences*. Cambridge University Press, Cambridge.

von Wright, G.H. (2004) *Explanation and Understanding*. Cornell University Press, Ithaca, NY.

9. *Dignity as an Object of Empirical Study: Experiences from Two Research Programmes*

Lennart Nordenfelt

9.1 General considerations

The results of the empirical studies in the two projects focused upon in this book, the Home project and the DOE project (Dignity and Older Europeans) are very rich. The country teams have collected an impressive volume of material which it will take a long time to analyse thoroughly. As will have become evident already, it is easy to give examples of quality of life, autonomy, integrity and dignity from the various studies in the two projects. This holds in particular for quality of life and autonomy in the Home project and for dignity in the DOE project. Dignity was the target concept in the DOE project, whereas good care in a broad sense was the target concept in the Home project.

9.1.1 Background
There is a major theoretical problem in research projects in which conceptual analysis encounters empirical studies where the standard terms that connote the concepts under scrutiny, such as the terms 'quality of life', 'satisfaction', 'autonomy', 'integrity' and 'dignity', are used by ordinary native speakers. One aspect of this problem is illustrated by the Slovak woman (in the DOE project; see Chapter 1) who wondered why we asked about dignity in care. Dignity, she says, is not an ordinary word: it is a word used by priests.

The purpose of philosophical conceptual analysis is never simply to map ordinary language in all its bewildering variety. The analysis must contain a crucial element of reconstruction and even stipulation, although the intention can vary in this respect. One purpose of a conceptual analysis, as I see it, is to improve on ordinary language. It must entail an element of clarification and specificity. The result of a good conceptual analysis should be a map of a series of concepts that is simpler and more fruitful for further communication than the initial complicated and sometimes even inconsistent map that may be the immediate result of an empirical study. In the two introductory chapters of this book I have attempted to create a slightly idealised map, where some of the crucial relations between the concepts will, I hope, have become clearer.

It is not the task of lay people who are approached by researchers to take part in such a conceptual analysis. They answer concrete questions and in their answers they use such terms as they find adequate to express their thoughts. Often they use their own spontaneous language. In some instances, however, the language of the respondents has been influenced by the interviewer. This is particularly salient in the DOE project with its heavy emphasis on questions about dignity.

On the other hand, a conceptual analysis need not be paralysed by the use of specific terms. It may become clear that there exists a salient notion of dignity, for instance, without a specific term being used by the respondents. None of the older people interviewed in the DOE project mentioned the learned term *Menschenwürde*. However, almost all of them expressed the basic idea that human beings possess an innate dignity. Some participants, especially those from countries with a strong religious tradition, thought that this innate dignity signified humanity's divine origin, while others merely accepted its existence. In all countries the notions associated with this type of dignity were human rights, autonomy and equality. And the participants maintained that a minimum level of dignity is attached to all persons.

Similar observations were made regarding the other types of dignity in the model that has been proposed here. This proves that the model may be used as a tool for analysis. The dignity of merit was mentioned (although in other terms). It occurred in discussion about positions in society as well as when the wisdom of older people was at issue. The discussion about rank and position often concerned health professionals, especially doctors, whose rank and dignity have traditionally been high in many European countries. However, as the discussion among UK respondents reveals, many professionals have lost this kind of dignity because of high-profile cases of misconduct and neglect.

The dignity of moral stature came up in different ways in different countries. In Spain and Slovakia it came up frequently, especially when older people remarked on the need to regain respect from others. In order to acquire such respect, they said, one had to behave correctly and respect their rights. Certain virtues that older people require to live well were also mentioned. These included the courage to face some of the adverse effects of ageing and the determination to retain independence during old age. Many people thought that moral standards in these respects were falling, and this meant reduction in the trust that they had in those around them.

The dignity of identity (represented by such aspects as feelings of identity, autonomy, integrity, inclusion in a community, self-confidence, self-respect and self-esteem) was of the utmost importance to many participants. It was particularly emphasised by many of the older people in Europe that they should be recognised as individuals with a history and with hopes and desires for the future.

9.1.2 A discussion of some problematic cases

In the DOE project, the four-notion model of dignity (Nordenfelt 2004) was explicitly challenged in some cases. The British team, for instance, remarked that some of the examples and some of the concepts mentioned by the respondents in the context of dignity did not fit the four-notion model. They highlighted in particular the concepts of trust, pride and loneliness. Trust was regarded as important in order to have and feel dignity. And with regard to pride one participant said:

We were brought up to care for ourselves, to take pride in our appearance. And I think dignity is a personal thing [*that has to do with this*] (UK, Dignity of Older Europeans/Older People, p. 42).

I think there are three major interpretations here, which may all be in accordance with the four-notion model. Two of them entail that trust and pride are important for dignity without being part of the sense of dignity. The third interpretation entails that they belong to the sense of dignity. In all cases I think that the dignity of identity is the most natural choice of dignity from our model. But it could also be the dignity of merit.

- Interpretation 1: Trust and pride enhance the dignity of identity.
- Interpretation 2: Trust and pride are signs that the dignity of identity exists.
- Interpretation 3: Trust and pride are parts of one's dignity of identity.

All, I think, are plausible interpretations. Trust is the opposite of fear of threats. When one fears that one's body or one's self is threatened, then it is one's identity that is threatened. In some cases one can certainly also fear that one's position or rank is threatened. Hence in this case the dignity of merit is involved. When one is proud one is proud of something that belongs to one's person, for instance one's body and self; but one can certainly also be proud of achievements and of a specific position in life.

Loneliness, finally, is a notion that I think is clearly related to the dignity of identity. In my initial presentation of the concept I explicitly identified inclusion in a community as a part of one's identity.

The French team made an interesting distinction that may be specific to the French language (France, Dignity of Older Europeans/Older People, p. 9). They distinguish between *having no dignity (indignité)* and *losing one's dignity (perte de dignité)*. Having no dignity is related to amoral behaviour. A person who is abusing someone else does not have any dignity. This exemplifies clearly the dignity of moral stature. But one can lose one's dignity (*perdre sa dignité*) through external events and through illness and loss of autonomy. Thus this expression illustrates the dignity of identity.

The French also seem to make a clear distinction between using the term 'dignity' about oneself (the subjective view) and about someone else (the objective view). Again the subjective view is more concerned with moral stature, but also willpower and control. The objective view concerns good appearance, suitable behaviour and showing positive feelings. These distinctions were not acknowledged in the other languages.

9.1.3 The distinction between quality of life and dignity again

In the Slovak presentation (Slovakia, Dignity of Older Europeans/Older People) the following significant sentences have a central place: 'Satisfaction with life appeared to be key in relation to experiencing dignity in the lives of these older people' and: 'Inner contentment appeared to participants to be an expression of dignity' (pp. 10, 12). The question to be asked here is: Do these informants genuinely consider dignity (in one of its senses) to be identical with subjective quality of life or satisfaction with life? Or is there a risk that we as interpreters wrongly come to this conclusion?

As I have argued before in the theoretical analysis, there is a more plausible interpretation. Satisfaction with life may be a sign that dignity is there, without this satisfaction with life being identical with or constituting dignity. Moreover, the results show that the relevant satisfaction concerns life in general. People do not refer to any old pleasure or just a good laugh and say that it is dignity-related. The feeling of dignity seems to be a feeling about an enduring state of affairs related to one's person. This feeling leads to or involves some satisfaction with life. Such an interpretation is plausible and does not contradict the theoretical model.

9.2 Basic ethical concepts: a comparison between the DOE project and the Home project

9.2.1 Introduction

Whereas the DOE project was designed around the specific concept of dignity, the Home project has had a much more varied connection with the basic ethical concepts scrutinised in this book. The Home project has had four main sub-projects:

1 The concepts of home, autonomy, dignity and quality of life (mainly a theoretical study).
2 What are the important values towards the end of life for older people themselves and their relatives in different settings of care?
3 Negotiations before death – the significance of cultural diversity at the end of life in one's own home.
4 The significance of good care in their family home for people with dementia.

In particular sub-projects 2 and 4, but also to some extent 3, have centred around the good care of older people either in their own homes or in residential homes. In the description of good care several of the basic concepts in this book have been highlighted. Terms such as 'satisfaction', 'quality of life', 'preservation of autonomy', 'integrity' and 'dignity' have been used. Only one of the specific studies in sub-project 2, that of Franklin et al. (2006), focused particularly on dignity and its preservation.

The good care of older people as identified in the Home project, however, is often characterised in terms similar to what is called 'dignified care' in some of the DOE studies. It can therefore be enlightening to compare the results from the two main projects in this respect. A particularly useful starting point is provided by the French team in the DOE project.

9.2.2 The idea of good or dignified care according to the DOE project

The idea of dignified care – carried out by professionals – as an action entailing paying respect to the dignity of the older person was a topic in all DOE reports. However, it is not always explicitly and clearly acknowledged. In one of the French reports it is particularly salient. The French group (DOE, France, Professionals, p. 36) provide an explicit list of examples of 'treating a person with dignity':

1 Preserving the social standing of a person
2 Giving personalised support
3 Making the person feel that they are of value

Table 9.1 Dignities to be preserved or enhanced

1	Social standing	Dignity of merit, dignity of identity
2	Personalised support	Dignity of identity
3	Being of value	Human dignity, dignity of merit, dignity of identity
4	Autonomy	Human dignity, dignity of identity
5	Habits	Dignity of identity
6	Home and privacy	Human dignity, dignity of identity
7	Comfort	Dignity of identity
8	Necessary care	Human dignity, dignity of identity
9	Agreement/consent	Human dignity, dignity of identity, in particular autonomy
10	Power of decision	Dignity of identity, in particular autonomy
11	Avoidance of separation	Dignity of identity
12	Cleanliness	Dignity of identity
13	Preservation of morality	Dignity of moral stature
14	Avoidance of humiliation	Dignity of identity

4   Supporting and maintaining autonomy
5   Respecting the individual's habits and keeping things as they like them
6   Respecting their home and privacy
7   Giving comfort in living
8   Giving the necessary care
9   Asking for agreement/consent for the care to be given
10 Letting the power of decision in care and in the choice of home be with the old person
11 Not separating or isolating them from life
12 Keeping the person clean
13 Not letting a person transgress social or moral laws, i.e. protect them
14 Not putting a person in a position of failure in a group.

It is of interest to consider what are the dignities to be preserved or enhanced here. Table 9.1 shows my suggestions (the dignities mentioned sometimes occur together, and sometimes they are alternatives).

9.2.3   The Home project and the values to be enhanced in good care

The Home project contains several analyses of values in the good care of older people and, in particular, in the care at the end of the patient's life. In a number of papers the Swedish nursing scientists Ternestedt, Rinell Hermansson and colleagues have provided a theoretical framework for good terminal care and made empirical studies of end-of-life care. Rinell Hermansson et al. (2000) and Ternestedt et al. (2002) are inspired by an analysis of good terminal care which was performed by Weisman & Kastenbaum (1968) and Weisman (1972) in developing a nursing model of the care of dying patients. This model is based on six crucial questions that should determine whether or not a deceased person has had an appropriate death.

- Did the patient have adequate medical care and relief from pain towards the end of their life?
- How completely did the patient manage their life up until the time of death?
- To what degree did the patient maintain rewarding or significant relationships during the terminal period?
- Did the patient die with a decent self-image and a feeling of personal significance?
- Were there signs of conflict resolution?
- Was there a 'personal consent to die' – in that the patient had nothing more to live for?

On the basis of these questions Ternestedt et al. (2002) propose a conceptual frame-work for the evaluation of end-of-life nursing care. This framework contains as a kernel six keywords which, conveniently for pedagogic purposes, all start with the letter S:

- *Symptom control* concerns optimal alleviation of symptoms based on the individual patient's needs and wishes.
- *Self-determination* concerns the support of the patient so that he or she is as optimally involved in the care as possible.
- *Social relationships* concern the support of the patient in maintaining important social relationships and in meeting relatives and friends.
- *Self-image* concerns the patient's self-description and his or her outlook and lifestyle.
- *Synthesis and summation* concern supporting the patient in creating and seeing continuity and meaning in life.
- *Surrender*, finally, concerns how to support the patient in accepting that death is imminent.

With the help of these six S keywords, Ternestedt et al. provide an *a priori* list of values (see Chapter 7). Other members of the Home project have attempted to extract basic values in the care of older or dying people through interview studies. Wallgren (2002) and Arama (2002) have interviewed providers and patients about values to be enhanced in good care of older people and have as a result compiled lists of such values. Österlind (2002) and Karlsson (2003), although they partly have a different focus, also contribute to the summation of values. The components of these catalogues of values are often similar to the items on the French list of factors enhancing dignity from the DOE project (see above).

The authors within the Home project rarely use the language of dignity but instead present the relevant values as elements or results of good care in general. The focus in Wallgren's study is on how treatment and care in the patient's own home can enhance these values. The study was performed at a unit for advanced home care services. Such services are mainly delivered to patients who are terminally ill, often in the late stages of cancer. Wallgren interviewed the care providers. Arama studied palliative home care but focused on the patient's perspective by actually interviewing patients, who were all in receipt of hospital-affiliated palliative home care. Österlind studied the care culture within special residential homes for the care of older people, interviewing staff members. Karlsson, finally, primarily investigated the views of nurses and other staff on the factor of ethnicity in the palliative care of older people.

Freedom of choice, autonomy and participation

Care in their own home was found to promote the patients' freedom of choice. They had more freedom to abstain from treatment or specialised care, or to take part in treatment or care decisions. They were also more inclined to make decisions about their care and participate in the care when they were treated at home than when they were treated in an institution. It was also emphasised that the patients had a greater opportunity to choose which nurse to have the closest contact with.

> *Patients have a stronger patient role in their homes than in the institutions. Here they are in their own homes ... everything is theirs, so we come in as guests* (Swedish home-care nurse in the Home project, Wallgren 2002, p. 18. The translations from Swedish in this quotation and below are my own)

> *I can do what I want ... I can dress and go out and can lie down to read or do a crossword. I can make a pancake when I feel like it ... I can do whatever I want* (Swedish female patient in the Home project, Arama 2002, p. 16).

Freedom of choice and autonomy are also highlighted as a value in the institutional setting:

> *A meaningful day is to let the individual do what he or she wants. To respect that the residents don't always want to take part in general activities* (Swedish member of a palliative care team in the Home project, Österlind 2002, p. 26).

Preserved integrity

Nurses mentioned that the patients appreciated the opportunity to preserve their integrity in their own homes. The home was a stable and well-known place in their life. The patients decided how things were to be in their homes with regard to care, and they were allowed to do so by the health-care personnel. As a consequence they felt stronger in defending other elements of their privacy. A nurse expresses this as follows:

> *One has to sense what one is allowed to do here, one cannot just intrude into the home. One has to meet the patient and the relatives where they are ... one cannot take away the hope, but one must also tell them, it is difficult not to tread on their toes ... not to cross the border and all this is more important in a home* (Swedish nurse in the Home project, Wallgren 2002, p. 21).

> *I think they want to be cared for at home because the hospital setting is not very friendly. It is stressful, it is noisy and it is difficult to get any help* (Swedish nurse in the Home project, Karlsson 2003, p. 15).

Availability of care

The patients receiving palliative care at home are completely dependent on getting help from health-care professionals almost immediately. The availability of health-care professionals is therefore ranked as a high value by most patients.

Participation of relatives
It is evident that relatives play a great role in home care. It is very common for a relative, often a spouse, to lives at home together with the patient. The relative is normally active in the day-to-day care and is naturally deeply interested and involved in the medical treatment of the patient. Health care in the patient's own home makes this possible.

Enhanced communication; deeper contacts
Being in the home environment creates other possibilities for open and intimate communication. The nurse can also more easily adapt information to the individual patient and their situation. The nurse is also immediately informed about the patient's total life situation. Moreover, being at home strengthens the patient's self-confidence and encourages them to pose questions to which they need an answer.

> *Good care for me is that those who come to my home listen to me and take me seriously, and if I ask for advice that they give good advice* (patient in the Home project, Arama 2002, p. 28).

> *When one is at home with a patient ... it is always quiet, one is rarely so stressed that one cannot sit down in peace and quiet and have a conversation. This is prioritised in a different way [in the home]* (Swedish nurse in the Home project, Wallgren 2002, p. 23).

The patient is seen in their social context
This follows from what has been said about communication and contacts. The fact that nurses enter the patient's home also means that they get to know about the physical setting within which the patient lives and can act accordingly.

Feeling of security
The home is (normally) an environment that the patient likes a lot and is well acquainted with. It contributes to a feeling of security. The home also normally contributes to a comfortable life and a chance to pursue one's ordinary life as much as possible.

Sense of community; closeness to other people
As well as the spouses or other relatives of the patients who function as co-carers, the respondents mention that the home also provides more opportunities for contact with other significant people, such as friends and neighbours. Many older people find such contacts highly rewarding.

The home provides aesthetic values
In many instances patients have invested much time and energy into designing their homes according to their own aesthetic tastes. An institution rarely has similar aesthetic qualities. To be in surroundings that you find beautiful certainly enhances your well-being.

The patient study (Arama 2002) highlighted some further points, mainly to do with the *patient–carer encounter*. The quality of this encounter, Arama summarises, depends on the basic attitude of the carer, their ability to be present in the moment, ability to

197

show warmth and closeness and at the same time keep a distance according to the situation.

I don't think one can compare being in a hospital with home care. Home care comes much closer and in the hospital there are so many routines. They are in a hurry, I am afraid (patient in the Home project, Arama 2002, p. 22).

One can feel the fantastic warmth and love and that is very important to us who have a disease like this (patient in the Home project, Arama 2002, p. 23).

Empathy, that one feels that it is sincere, that this person is really interested in me and cares for me. That's what is most important. Then it does no harm if the person is clever too (patient in the Home project, Arama 2002, p. 25).

Karlsson (2005a) highlights the *holistic* aim of palliative care – which has been present but not made particularly explicit in the previous studies. The holistic ideology entails that the carer should consider the patient as a whole, integrated person. From an ethical point of view this is already included in the concept of respect for the person. But there is also a scientific element crucial to adequate care. Since a person is an integrated whole consisting of physical, mental and social aspects, and since these aspects interact, one should be open to the fact that a physical ailment can have a psychological or social origin or vice versa. This aim, however, is in general not well taken care of in traditional palliative care. Karlsson quotes a consultant physician who says:

90% of what we do concerns physical aspects. 10% concerns the mental and the rest receives no attention from us. This is the case at least for doctors (Swedish geriatrician in the Home project, Karlsson 2003, p. 13).

Some of the nurses also complain:

We sometimes talk with people about their quality of life, but this is not always documented (Swedish palliative care nurse in the Home project, Karlsson 2003, p. 13).

9.2.4 Comparison between the French and Swedish lists of elements of good care

As I noted in section 9.2.2 above, the French DOE report provided a list of examples of treating a person with dignity. Comparing this list with the findings of the Swedish Home project with regard to good care, one can find crucial overlaps. The following items are shared (the six S key concepts are shown in italics):

1 Supporting and maintaining autonomy, including asking for agreement/consent for the care and letting the power of decision be with the old person (*self-determination*)
2 Respecting the patient's home and privacy (integrity) (*self-determination, self-image*)
3 Giving personalised support and respecting the individual's habits (*self-image*)
4 Giving comfort in living (*synthesis and summation*)
5 Not separating or isolating them from life (*social relationships*)
6 Giving the necessary care and keeping the person clean (which is not explicitly stated but taken for granted in the Swedish empirical studies) (*symptom control*).

One interesting difference between the French and the Swedish studies is that the Swedish respondents emphasise the *quality of the encounter* and the *depth of communication*. The Swedish patients also value particularly highly *availability* and a *feeling of security*.

A striking item in the French list that has no counterpart in the Swedish studies is the one about not letting the patient transgress social or moral laws, although this has little relevance when we are dealing with the care of the terminally ill. However, it should be kept in mind all along that there are two different categories of patients in the two projects: older people, mainly in nursing homes, in the DOE project and seriously or even terminally ill people, mainly in their own homes but sometimes in nursing homes, in the Home project.

A further comparison can be made between the findings in the two projects and the characterisation of good palliative care given by the World Health Organization (WHO 2005):

Palliative care is an approach which improves the quality of life of patients and their families facing life-threatening illness, through the prevention, assessment and treatment of pain and other physical, psychological and spiritual problems.

Palliative care:

- Provides relief from pain and other distressing symptoms
- Affirms life and regards dying as a normal process
- Intends neither to hasten nor postpone death
- Integrates the psychological and spiritual aspects of patient care
- Offers a support system to help patients live as actively as possible until death
- Offers a support system to help the family cope during the patient's illness and in their own bereavement
- Uses a team approach to address the needs of patients and their families, including bereavement counselling, if indicated
- Will enhance quality of life, and may also positively influence the course of illness.

WHO is explicit about pain relief, comfort and support. It is also explicit about support of the family. But again the aspects of communication and close human contact are not highlighted.

9.2.5 Patients on the edge of life

It is interesting to compare the findings of the DOE project and the Home project with the results of a recent doctoral dissertation on the life situation of critically ill or even dying patients in nursing homes in Norway (Hov 2007). The dissertation also analyses what constitutes good nursing of people in this kind of situation. One of Hov's main findings was that the situation of the patients was hard and burdensome. Four themes were emphasised:

- *Waiting in confusion* meant that the patients were left waiting for clarification of the goals of their treatments.

- *Loneliness* meant that the patients by and large felt quite lonely (care staff seldom talked to them about their situation).
- *Exhausted through suffering* meant that the patients were often troubled by problems with pain, breathing and vomiting.
- *Loss of control and agency* meant that the patients were totally in the power of other people and were seldom able to ask for or refuse help (p. 22).

Accordingly, the patients have a number of needs summarised by Hov. They have a need for *preparedness*, i.e. they need to be prepared for what is coming, and to be *free from mental suffering* and manage to keep their *hopes* up. They have a need for *human relations*, they need to meet people and not be abandoned. Finally, they have a need for *comfort, pain relief and security*.

Hov talks about the critically ill patient's need for *dignity* as the overall need, without making an explicit analysis of the concept of dignity. However, she describes the essential components of good nursing care, i.e. the kind of care that should meet the patient's need for dignity, in the following way:

> Good nursing care for these patients in nursing homes was captured as *meeting the patient's need for dignity*, illuminating what good nursing care could attain, and what could happen when nursing care was inadequate. ... Nursing care was conceived to contribute to *reconciliation* for the patient, depending on variations in the care in relation to how well the patient's wishes and needs were expressed, interpreted and followed. It was also related to the staff's communication with the patient about his/her situation and existential questions. When the care took as its starting point the patient's wishes this could help the patient to get hold of reality and talk about meaning, hope and religious needs. (pp. 23–24)

Many elements in Hov's findings correspond to the results from the DOE and Home projects. This holds for symptom control, comfort and general support. Hov also underlines the patient's need for human contact and opportunity to discuss existential questions. What is significant about Hov's findings, which mirrors the fact that her patients were critically ill or dying, is that the element of confusion can be great, and there may be a great loss of control as well as mental suffering and despair in the face of imminent death.

9.3 Salient aspects of the care of seriously ill older people in the Swedish context

9.3.1 Importance of human contacts and relations
Three studies in the Home project (Österlind 2002; Franklin et al. 2006; Hellström et al. 2005, 2007) especially address the importance of human relations among older people. The three studies, however, have quite different foci. Österlind investigated special residential homes for older people and conducted focus group interviews with the staff; Franklin interviewed 12 old and sick patients in two nursing homes; and Hellström studied the lives of 20 couples where one of the spouses had increasing dementia. (In this case the source of information was interviews with both spouses.)

Österlind noted that loneliness is a significant factor among the older people living in residential homes. This is noteworthy, since the possibility of human contact is one of the arguments for choosing a residential home instead of staying in one's own home. But as the informants say:

There is great loneliness among many people.

And:

They don't know each other, so it is not easy for them to talk (members of staff, Österlind 2002, p. 24).

Franklin et al. (2006), who studied very ill older people, underline their loneliness. If a person has little or no external contact, the loneliness can become extremely depressing. On the other hand, supportive attitudes on the part of both staff and next to kin seemed to help strengthen these older patients.

I have a family with grandchildren and that is nice. I don't see them often but my husband comes to see me almost every day (old Swedish woman in a nursing home, Franklin et al. 2006, p. 140).

Immigrant professionals were struck by the fact that older people in Sweden appeared to be so lonely. In these professionals' own cultures this would have been unheard of. Families, including the oldest generation, generally live together and their fate is shared. This impression is highlighted by Karlsson (2003), who pays particular attention to the role of ethnicity in the care of older people.

Instead of seeing your old mum as a weak and sick person, in other countries you would say that mum who is so well must come home now. Here we have a lot to learn from immigrants (Swedish nurse in the Home project, Karlsson 2003, p. 20).

9.3.2 The good death – the dignified death

In a few of the studies, in particular that of Österlind (2002), a special section is devoted to the good death. It is striking that this is a context where the word 'dignity' is mentioned spontaneously by the informants. People talk in a natural way about 'dignified death' or 'dying with dignity'.

There are two possible interpretations of such expressions. One has to do with the agency of the dying person themself. Here the dying person shows fortitude and courage in facing their imminent fate and behaves in a composed way. This would be an example of dignity of moral stature. According to the other, and perhaps more common interpretation, the dying person is looked upon as a patient, who should be treated and cared for with respect for their dignity. We are then talking about the person's dignity of identity or human dignity (*Menschenwürde*).

Österlind's informants mainly have the second interpretation in mind.

... It is dignity, I think, to be treated in a peaceful and professional way and to be liberated from pain (Swedish nurse in the Home project, Österlind 2002, p. 29).

The value of couplehood

Hellström et al. (2005, 2007) focused specifically on couples living together in their own homes. A criterion of inclusion in the study was that one member of the couple had increasing dementia, with the spouse having a central role in the daily care of the demented person. In one of Hellström's case studies a particular couple, Mr and Mrs Svensson (as she calls them), are studied closely. Mrs Svensson has dementia. The two have lived together for a long time, and Mr Svensson constantly emphasised how their relationship was genuinely reciprocal and life-enhancing for them both. He demonstrated a remarkable sensitivity to the needs of his spouse and provided assistance in a very thoughtful way.

A lot of things are important [in life]. I believe in God and we have a mutual belief and spend a lot of time in church. ... It is also lovely having a partner, to be able to help each other ... I also have a sister and brothers and relatives and we get around a lot (Mr Svensson in the Home project, Hellström et al., 2005, p. 16).

It was a general observation in Hellström's study that close and rewarding pair bond was extremely significant for the quality of life of both partners, not just the demented person. In addition to good communication many of the relationships were characterised by bonds of affection. Both partners worked hard to maintain these bonds. Hellström found that there were three factors that tended to ensure the quality of life and the quality of the relationship between the partners: enjoying life's little pleasures, continuous searching for positive aspects and living for today.

Do you think about the future? That is the last thing I do. I take each day as it comes. There is no reason to worry (old person with dementia in the Home project, Hellström et al., 2007, p. 396).

In one study, Hellström et al. (2007) make use of the expression 'doing things together'. When the two spouses can indeed work together, for instance in cooking, baking or gardening, their relationship becomes particularly rewarding. They can then support each other's self-esteem by building on residual strengths and affirming rather than compromising their efforts.

I mean, it works very well. She does the laundry and ironing, we clean together. I vacuum and she dusts, so it works well, and then we go shopping together as much as we can, otherwise I go myself. It depends on how much she has got to do at home (husband of a demented Swedish woman, Hellström et al., 2007, p. 400).

9.3.3 Significance of culture in the good care of older people

In a series of papers, Karlsson (2003, 2005a, 2005b) has focused on the care of terminally ill immigrants in the Swedish health-care system. Her observations and interviews are related to a special unit for palliative home care in the Stockholm area. Practically all the patients have some form of cancer in what is considered to be a terminal stage. Several, but not all, of the patients have a non-Swedish, often non-European, origin.

Karlsson notes that there are differences in the attitudes of the Swedish nurses towards Swedish and non-Swedish patients. These differences follow a hidden hierarchy according to which the relevant nationalities are ranked. Scandinavian immigrants are treated almost as if they were Swedish, whereas people from countries further away come lower down in the hierarchy. The hierarchy does not simply depend on geographical distance: the cultural, not least the religious, distance is crucial.

The situation is ambivalent, however. The nurses are often quite conscious of nursing ideals with regard to the caring encounter, says Karlsson (2005a). Indeed, they express the opinion that they should have the same attitude towards immigrant patients as towards Swedish patients in similar situations. They maintain that people should be approached from the point of view of their individual personalities and their individual needs and wishes. On the other hand, when immigrant patients are considered in the care situation their individual differences are often assessed within their specific cultural framework. For instance, the individual features of the immigrants are often explained in terms of their national origin or their religious affiliation. This is rarely the case with the Swedish patients. It is not considered relevant to explain an aspect pertaining to a Swedish patient with reference, for instance, to the fact that this patient comes from a particular region of Sweden or that they are Catholic. Thus, according to these nurses, Swedes have individual differences that do not need to be explained, whereas immigrants have individual differences that can be explained to a great extent by cultural factors.

Evidently there is a risk that immigrant patients, in particular those from distant origins, will be judged according to a stereotyped pattern. Paradoxically, the prejudices about the stereotype may be reinforced when the health-care staff pursue further studies about foreign cultures. If the cultural studies have only a modest ambition – which is the most plausible scenario in a standard education for doctors, nurses and nursing assistants – then the impression can be conveyed that the specific cultural features are more universally applicable than they in fact are. This observation, however, is of course no argument for abstaining from disseminating cultural knowledge. It only underlines the importance of placing cultural knowledge in context. Arabs, for instance, are as individual as Swedes. But it may be useful to know that a great number of Muslim Arabs follow the dicta of the Koran on particular occasions, for instance when decisions on family matters or financial affairs have to be made.

A specific situation where culture may play a role, but where prejudices may also confuse, is when the care staff have to decide whether to tell a patient and their relatives about the diagnosis and prognosis of the patient's disease. Karlsson (2005a) refers to a case where a male nurse discusses a patient from Turkey.

The typical situation in a Turkish family, if we take that example, is that the relatives tell the nurse what should and should not be said. It is not the sick person who makes this decision. You rarely encounter this with Swedish families. What might happen there is that the sick person him or herself says: 'I don't want to know, I don't want to be informed', but it is not common that the family does so (Swedish nurse in the Home project, Karlsson 2005a, p. 306).

The same nurse complicates this picture, however. He mentions a discussion about an information pamphlet that was to be issued by the palliative care centre. In this brochure it was stated that 'the care at the palliative care unit deals with the mitigation of symptoms where cure is no longer possible.' Some relatives of patients involved in the palliative care, as well as some patients themselves, reacted vehemently to this wording.

People thought, you shouldn't say this. This concerned both patients and relatives. So we have removed this wording from the new information material (Swedish nurse in the Home project, Karlsson 2005a, p. 306).

9.4   Conclusions

The two projects referred to in this book – the DOE project and the Home project – have in their various ways explored the notion of the good life for, as well as the good care of, people who are old and often sick or disabled. The Home project considered the good life and the good care in general quality-of-life terms, whereas the DOE project focused on the conditions for preserving and restoring a person's dignity. The different research emphases have in part yielded different results but there are several conclusions that are common to the two projects.

Perhaps contrary to what one might have expected, the notion of dignity appeared to be important to most ordinary people. Many had a feeling for the concept and could relate to at least some of the types of dignity in the four-notion model. This was particularly salient with human dignity and dignity of identity. But the dignity of merit and dignity of moral stature also raised important issues, especially for many professionals. As Tadd & Calnan (this volume, Chapter 6) observe:

These participants indicated that working with older people is not regarded as highly as working in other specialties. ... Professionals also reported their frustration at being unable to live up to the moral and professional requirements of their role, due to lack of resources, understaffing or inadequate care environments.

It was also clear that many older people think that for the most part they are not treated with dignity, either by members of society in general or by the care staff in residential homes. These older people often feel that they are either completely ignored or looked down upon. Partly as a result of this, they are often left in great loneliness. Those who are living in residential homes because of illness or disability often report decent medical care and symptom control, but at the same time neglect and indifference with regard to their social and existential needs. The studies from the Home project come to similar conclusions although they mostly characterise the care and treatment of older people not as violations of dignity but rather as deviations from the ideal of good care.

In this chapter I have observed how the requirements regarding dignity (as formulated by the French DOE group) coincide to a great extent with the definition of good care made in the Home project. The most salient overlapping items can be summarised as follows:

- Supporting and maintaining autonomy
- Respecting the patient's home and privacy
- Giving personalised support
- Giving comfort in living
- Upholding social relations
- Giving the necessary care.

References

Arama, K. (2002) Fenomenet vård i det egna hemmet, som det upplevs av patienter [The phenomenon of care in private homes as it is experienced by patients]. Master's thesis, Department of Caring Science, Ersta Sköndal University College, Stockholm.

Dignity and Older Europeans (2004) Final Report of Focus Groups (2002–2004) http://www.cardiff.ac.uk/dignity.

Franklin, L.-L., Ternestedt, B.-M. & Nordenfelt, L. (2006) Views on dignity of elderly nursing home residents. *Nursing Ethics*, **13**, 130–146.

Hellström, I., Nolan, M. & Lundh, U. (2005) We do things together: A case study of couple-hood. *Dementia: The International Journal of Social Research and Practice*, **4**, 7–22.

Hellström, I., Nolan, M. & Lundh, U. (2007) Sustaining 'couplehood'. Spouses' strategies for living positively with dementia. *Dementia: The International Journal of Social Research and Practice*, **6**, 383–409.

Hov, R. (2007) Nursing Care for Patients on the Edge of Life. PhD thesis, Karlstad University Studies 2007:33, Karlstad.

Karlsson, E. (2003) Det här skulle vara extremt ovanligt i en svensk familj [This would be extremely unusual in a Swedish family]. Master's thesis, Department of Ethnology, Stockholm University, Stockholm.

Karlsson, E. (2005a) Möten med Bahar. Om kultur och etnicitet vid vård i livets slutskede [Encounters with Bahar. On culture and ethnicity at the end of life] In: *Bruket av kultur. Hur kultur används och görs socialt verksamt* (ed M. Öhlander) pp. 295–314. Studentlitteratur, Lund.

Karlsson, E. (2005b) Delaktighet – ett värde i vården [Participation – a value in health care]. Paper presented at the conference Kulturstudier i Sverige: nationell forskarkonferens 13–15 June 2005, arranged by ACSIS, Linköping university.

Nordenfelt, L. (2004) The varieties of dignity. *Health Care Analysis*, **12**, 69–81.

Österlind, J. (2002) Hemmet på hemmet [Home in the home: the carer and the cared for in sheltered living for the elderly]. Master's thesis, The Department of Caring Science, Ersta Sköndal University College, Stockholm.

Rinell Hermansson, A. & Ternestedt, B.-M. (2000) What do we know about the dying patient? Awareness as a means to improve palliative care. *Medicine and Law*, **19**, 335–344.

Ternestedt, B.-M., Andershed, B., Eriksson, M. & Johansson, I. (2002) A good death: Development of a nursing model of care. *Journal of Hospice and Palliative Nursing*, **4**, 153–160.

Wallgren, E. (2002) Hemmets betydelse för den äldres upplevelse av god vård och död [The significance of the home for the experience of a good care and a good death among elderly persons]. Master's thesis, Department of Caring Science, Ersta Sköndal University College, Stockholm.

Weisman, A.D. (1972) *On Dying and Denying*. Behavioral Publications, New York.

Weisman, A.D. & Kastenbaum, R. (1968) *The Psychological Autopsy. A Study of the Terminal Phase of Life*. Community Mental Health Journal, Monograph **4**. Behavioral Publications, New York.

WHO (2005) *Palliative Care: What It Is*. http://www.who.int/cancer/palliative/en/

Index

ability
  cognitive 159; *see also* dementia
  first order 6–7
  loss of 93
  second order 5–7
abuse, in care 120
accountability, moral 35
act utilitarianism 180
action, freedom of 49
activity, moral 41
afterlife, belief in 152, 182–3
ageing, experience of 73–4
ageing body 5
  alienated 74
  experience of 73
ageism 130, 140, 147
agency 201
  loss of 200
alienation 54, 159
Alzheimer, A. 99
appearance 57
Aquinas, T. 183
Aristotle 9, 48
atheism 184
attributes, physical and mental 100
autonomy 18, right to 18, 20, 22, 39, 41, 48,
    92, 136, 141
  creation of 21, 22
  respect for 18, 22
  restricted 37
  violation of 19, 20
  see also choice; decision-making

Bauman, Z. 154
behaviour, ethical 71, 72
body
  as container 54

exposed in intimate care 134, 140
  objective 54–5
  personal 54
body–self 69–73
  conflict between 73
body–world encounter 69
brain death 72, 175
  see also dead; death
brutalisation 120
burdensomeness, fear of in old age 130–1

care 182
  availability 196, 199
  choice 136–7
  dignified 193–4
  emotional 138
  end-of-life 162, 195
  holistic 148
  individualised 158, 160
  intimate 134, 140
  low status of 128, 129; *see also* carers,
      morale
  person-centred 101
  personalised 138
  planning 150–1, 161
  routine 138
carer–patient encounter 197–8
carers
  dignity of 141
  job satisfaction 99, 128–9
  moral stature of 46
  morale of 120, 128
  stress experienced by 99
change, psychological 174
choice 10, 196
Christian anthropology 171
Christian morality 40

207